# IN SEARCH OF
# THE MODERN
# HIPPOCRATES

# IN SEARCH OF THE MODERN HIPPOCRATES

### EDITED BY
### ROGER J. BULGER

University of Iowa Press

Iowa City

University of Iowa Press, Iowa City 52242
Copyright © 1987 by the University of Iowa
All rights reserved
Printed in the United States of America
First edition, 1987

Book and jacket design by Patrick Hathcock
Typesetting by G & S Typesetters, Inc., Austin, Texas
Printing and binding by Braun-Brumfield, Inc., Ann Arbor, Michigan

Library of Congress Cataloging-in-Publication Data

In search of the modern Hippocrates.

   1. Medical ethics.   2. Physician and patient.
3. Healing.   I. Bulger, Roger J., 1933–
[DNLM: 1. Ethics, Medical. W 50 I35]
R724.I55   1987    174'.2    86-24950
ISBN 0-87745-160-5

*For Ruth and her Grace and Faith*

# Contents

## Part III. The Healing Context: Cultures, Persons, and Words

# Part IV. The Future for Physicianhood

# Acknowledgments

Gwen Clopton and Louise Milliner have provided invaluable support with the day-to-day details and complexities of organizing such a multi-authored book. It would never have happened without them. My thanks also must go to Drs. Griff Ross, Frank Webber, and Larry Grouse for their ideas, example, and friendly criticism.

A special note of thanks goes to Robert J. Glaser for his support in allowing four of these essays to be reprinted from *The Pharos*.

"The Golden Rule and the Cycle of Life" (chapter 5) by Erik H. Erikson is reprinted through the courtesy of the *Harvard Medical Alumni Bulletin* 37 (2), Winter 1963.

"Narcissus, Pogo, and Lewis Thomas' Wager" (chapter 6) by Roger J. Bulger is reprinted through the courtesy of the *Journal of the American Medical Association* 245 (14), April 1981.

"Emerging Unities of the Twenty-first Century" (chapter 8) by Roger J. Bulger is taken in part from and reprinted through the courtesies of the *Archives of Internal Medicine* 142, December 1982, and *The Pharos*, a publication of Alpha Omega Alpha Honor Medical Society, vol. 47 (2), Spring 1984.

"Words as Scalpels" (chapter 12) by Stanley J. Reiser is reprinted through the courtesy of the *Annals of Internal Medicine* 92 (6), June 1980.

"Placebos, Patients, and Physicians" (chapter 13) by Howard M. Spiro is reprinted through the courtesy of *The Pharos*, a publication of Alpha Omega Alpha Honor Medical Society, vol. 47 (2), Spring 1984.

"The Future of Medical Practice" (chapter 15) by Arnold S. Relman is reprinted through the courtesy of *Health Affairs* 2 (2), Summer 1983.

"Technology and the Eclipse of Individualism in Medicine" (chapter 16) by Stanley J. Reiser is reprinted through the courtesy of *The Pharos*, a publication of Alpha Omega Alpha Honor Medical Society, vol. 45 (1), Winter 1982.

"A Postscript from the Physician as Patient" (chapter 18) by David E. Rogers is reprinted through the courtesy of *The Pharos*, a publication of Alpha Omega Alpha Honor Medical Society, vol. 49 (3), Summer 1986.

# PART I.
## *The Need for Direction*

# 1. *The Modern Context for a Healing Profession*

**Roger J. Bulger**

The future of the profession of medicine in America is, at the very least, under serious question. Almost everything about the practice of medicine, the role of the physician, and the nature of the doctor-patient relationship is being reexamined critically. In fact, there are those who predict that in ten years we will not recognize the health care delivery enterprise. On the other hand, it is important to remember that the profession is still heavily influenced by its commitment to service as embodied in the ancient Oath of Hippocrates. In one sense this book is about the essential nature of this oath taking to the continued life of the medical profession and ends with an attempt at constructing a new oath which might adequately guide doctors in the years ahead.

The most striking societal characteristic of the past twenty years has been the accelerating rate of change we have experienced. In fact, people no longer are surprised by change; they expect it, and they are not upset by dramatic, sweeping alteration of a sort that a previous generation would have found devastating. The only thing that might startle us would be if nothing changed for a year or so.

Administrators two decades ago, if they wanted to be creative and different, aspired to be "change agents"; now it could be argued that, in the midst of changes everywhere, the most creative administrator might wish to be a "preservation agent," by which I mean someone who seeks to preserve essential values and hence essential elements of organizations, institutions, professions, and other subsets of society such that the baby is not thrown out with the bathwater in our efforts to adjust to an ever-changing environment.

Against this backdrop it is well to remember that good history cannot be written by active participants in events as those events unfold; a certain necessary perspective must be achieved before a proper interpretation and understanding of events can be developed. This creates a special problem for us these days when so much is happening so rapidly, and we all seem to know it. In earlier times, when important happenings occurred relatively infrequently, it was easier for citizens to know where they stood. Thus, all the current assessments of where our society is and is going, of where our health care delivery system is and is going, and of where the medical profession is and is going are themselves to be doubted. We must not and need not get lulled into a knee-jerk reflex of easy acceptance of all the latest trends and pressures; we need to remember that a journalist is not a historian.

We can affect what happens to ourselves, our organizations, our institutions, and our society in the future; and in fact we have an obligation to try to preserve what is best and what is essential to the core missions of our professions, agencies, or other societal subsets. It behooves all who care in a democratic society to listen to our social critics and observers, to be alert to possible futures, and to work for the development of the best of those futures.

With regard to medicine and its ongoing evolution and revolution, there is reason to worry about the future of the profession, the role of the doctor as healer, and, indeed, the profession's capacity to continue to attract to its ranks the brightest, most highly motivated, and most service-oriented of our youth. Will the medical-industrial complex destroy the physician as we know him or her by making the doctor an employee of a large profit-seeking corporation instead of the patient's prime advocate? Will the deregulation of the health industry turn the physician from the role of healer to that of a technology-purveying, cost-conscious businessperson trying to provide the best compromise between quality of product and profit margin? Or, more simply, will the continuing proliferation of technology make it quixotic to even aspire to sustain the nontechnological dimensions of the art of medicine and the

concept of the physician as healer? Will the continuing bureaucratiza-
tion of our modern society and its tendency to egalitarianism mean that
the effort to sustain a corps of elite people, with a special combination
of talents and commitments, is no longer viable? Will monetary concerns and the oft-touted surfeit of physicians destroy the profession by
discouraging the most able young people from entering it?

What merit can there be in searching for a modern Hippocrates? Why
should anyone be interested in defining and exploring the characteristics
and context of physicianhood? Haven't we all been treated to an excessive series of expositions in recent years on doctors and doctoring?
We've either unhorsed the Knight-Physician or we haven't; why not let
the subject drop?

My answer to the thrust of these queries is that the profession I love is
experiencing in this decade a kind of free-fall through a series of major
force fields, without any clear assurance that it won't be so reoriented by
these forces that it will miss the targeted safety net and, in effect, be
destroyed. American medicine has led the world; biomedical science has
spawned magnificently effective technologies which have in turn helped
to produce the most advanced and accessible health care in the world.
On the other hand, our system is expensive and has serious problems,
and there is much discontent with it. Enormous changes are under way
and there is the potential for future perturbations which could make
dramatic alterations in the nature of our enterprise. We all hope that the
changes will be positive for our society as a whole, for individual patients, and for the helping and healing professions; but it is equally
conceivable that in ten years social critics will be describing the golden
age of American medicine—by then no more—and world leadership
in yet another major area of human endeavor will have passed from our
hands. I regard the latter prospect as a sorry one and believe that the
loss of an elite corps of dedicated, highly educated, technically competent healers would be a major national cultural loss, one that should be
forestalled if at all possible.

The Japanese and the Chinese have, enmeshed in their cultural background and even in their language, the concept that a crisis is a threatening opportunity, and this book is dedicated to the premise that the crises
of the next decade can in fact produce an altered but strengthened and
improved medical profession. The powerful force fields referred to earlier include the incredible power of new technology, including the full
flowering of the computer in the practice of medicine; the growing appreciation of the chemistry of the brain and mind-body interactions; and
the emergence of the corporate scenario as the most likely theme in the
organization and financing of health care in the future. The net result of
all these is to exert tremendous pressure on the concept of physician-

hood. What is the core of being a doctor, when one is done stripping away this or that trapping or secondary characteristic? What are the essentials of physicianhood, which if they were to pass out of existence would take with them the whole profession, or at least that sturdy professional tree which has grown from the roots of Hippocrates?

Allow me briefly to enlarge on this thesis. As Stanley Reiser has so eloquently emphasized in recent years, new technology has the potential for a variety of effects on physician behavior and on the doctor-patient relationship. Historically, it can be shown that new technology can remove the physician in an ever-increasing fashion from intimate contact with the patient. We all worry that the computerization of medicine, both through the magic of new scans of various sorts and through the memory, evaluations, organization, and educational capacities of existing machines, will at last remove the physician from all but the most perfunctory of nontechnical interactions with the patient, making dehumanized, assembly-line, supermarket medicine an irrevocable reality. But Dr. Reiser says it need not be so; he thinks the doctor could use the computer to produce more time for listening to and talking with patients, paradoxically perhaps providing the technocrat doctor with the key resource to allow him or her to become a healing physician. This and related areas are explored by several contributors to this volume.

The burgeoning understanding of the working of the brain has opened up the exploration of mind-body interactions, allowing speculation and some analysis of the capacity for patients to heal themselves and for physicians to help them do so. Herbert Benson, an internist who has introduced and popularized the terms "the relaxation response" and "the faith factor," has been a pioneer in some of these areas and believes that an examination of the placebo effect can lead to new, more effective ways to mobilize the individual's own capacities to regain or sustain health. Confidence and trust in the physician on the part of the patient is essential to this dimension of healing, and it is the thesis here that this element of physicianhood, rather than being abandoned and denigrated as being nonspecific, should be studied, developed, and perfected by future physicians. Just as theoretical physics and theology/philosophy seem to be coming together, can it be that concepts of mind and body are intersecting and that scientific, western medicine can find its accommodations and points of contact with holistic medicine, religious healers, and some other heretofore strange approaches to health and disease? Attention is paid in several essays in this volume to the placebo effect, the use of the word in therapy, the nature of the trusting and therapeutic relationship, and the idea that we are experiencing the emergence of certain intellectual unities, a coming together of the arts and sciences and the reawakening of a sense of wonder at what we don't know and have still to learn.

Lastly, the pro-competition movement and all the activity that has entailed by both the public and private sectors, together with increased cost-consciousness on the part of purchasers (especially large group purchasers) of health care and the ramifications of the emerging oversupply of doctors, all combine, in the minds of some analysts, to produce an environment which will favor prospective capitation-based funding for the total health care of large groups of people. Serious predictions include the provision of health care by 1990 to half our population by perhaps twenty large firms which would employ physicians. Organized medicine may have escaped the specter of having its doctors on the payroll of "Big Brother" in the federal government, but, paradoxically, it may not have escaped the similar specter of the physician as an employee of a large bureaucratic corporation. Should employment slots become hard to find due to physician oversupply, will it be hard for the individual doctor to be the patient's advocate if his or her advocacy implies a higher cost and lower profitability for the firm? What will be his or her duty as a physician under such circumstances? If the corporate scenario does come true, can the essence of the physician's role as patient-advocate be preserved? If so, how should we do it? If most doctors are salaried, will they then unionize, as has happened elsewhere; and, if so, what will the impacts be on the society and the profession? If our physician excess becomes a broadly recognized fact, will there be or should there be an effort to bring our medicine to less fortunate people in foreign lands and are there dangers in the use of medicine as a diplomatic or foreign policy tool? These organizational, economic, and social trends all further underscore the need to clearly understand that essential core to physicianhood referred to earlier. We may ask whether in other westernized nations such changes have impacted negatively upon the essentials of the Hippocratic tradition.

In short, I believe that the next decade will be a major turning point for the profession of medicine in the United States. Each of the various forces now at play affecting health care has, in its own particular way, an effect upon the fundamental core relationship between doctor and patient. The essays presented in this volume are an attempt to address many of these issues, by no means in a comprehensive way and seldom from the same perspective, but always with an eye toward exposing the interested reader to the insights and perceptions of some of our wisest observers. Although the quality of that wisdom and of those insights may diminish in those pieces I produced, it is to be understood that these are included to bridge some obvious gaps and to introduce considerations not otherwise apparent in the other contributions. I am more hopeful now than I have ever been during the past twenty-five years of worried watching and anxious anticipation about the future of the medical profession that the rise of the modern Hippocrates is well under way and that there can be a health care system created which incorporates the answers to our most pressing societal problems without destroying the working space and context supportive of an individual human being dedicated to the return to health of other individual human beings. My attempt in the concluding essay to fashion a modern Hippocratic Oath is based on the firm conviction that the modern Hippocrates and his or her profession will more than ever need a compelling and meaningful covenant to guide activities which otherwise promise to become more complex, bureaucratic, and impersonal.

As I get older I am more and more impressed with the importance of the concept that a crisis is a threatening opportunity. For me, "The cup is half full" is a far more useful and creative observation than "The cup is half empty." In this effort to collect some wisdom and insight about our cup of medicine, I could have used the title *The End of the Hippocratic Tradition* but chose instead to call the book *In Search of the Modern Hippocrates*. There was really no contest, because I meet the modern disciples of Hippocrates in each new first-year medical school class and in each group of graduates. I'm distressed sometimes that they don't know who they are and don't fully appreciate the powers, limitations, and responsibilities of the medical mode, that they don't understand the values of the proud tradition they inherit, that they don't appreciate the breadth and depth of the unexplored opportunities before them, and that they aren't sufficiently alert to the dangers besetting the future of their profession. But I also remember that the same could have been said about me and many of my colleagues when we entered the profession twenty-five years ago. This collection of essays attempts to deal with these matters and is an effort to enlarge the reader's understanding of the possibilities for the modern Hippocrates and his and her patients. Our cup is only half full and we can fill it further if we will!

# 2. *The Search for a New Ideal*

Roger J. Bulger

> Life is short,
> The art long,
> Opportunity fleeting,
> Experiment treacherous,
> Judgement difficult.—Hippocrates, Aphorisms I

I will look upon him who shall have taught me this art even as one of my parents. I will share my substance with him, and I will supply his necessities, if he be in need. I will regard his offspring even as my own brethren and I will teach them this art, if they would learn it without fee or covenant. I will impart this art by precept, by lecture and by every mode of teaching, not only to my own sons but to sons of him who has taught me, and to disciples bound by covenant and oath, according to the law of medicine.

The regimen I adopt shall be for the benefit of my patients according to my ability and judgement, and not for their hurt or for any wrong. I will give no deadly drug to any, though it be asked of me, nor will I counsel such, and especially I will not aid a woman to procure abortion. Whatsoever house I enter, there will I go for the benefit of the sick, refraining from all wrongdoing or corruption, and especially from any act of seduction of male or female, of bond or free. Whatsoever things I see or hear concerning the life of men, in my attendance on the sick or even apart therefrom, which ought not to be noised abroad, I will keep silence thereon, counting such things to be as sacred secrets.—Hippocrates, Physician's Oath

These famous quotations of Hippocrates yield, upon careful examination, much wisdom, even for modern-day physicians. On the other hand, it is clear that the Hippocratic Oath contains some statements that are not, in fact, in agreement with what many, if not most, highly motivated and sincere twentieth-century physicians would hold. It may seem extraordinary that in all the time that has elapsed since the days of Hippocrates history has been unable to produce a statement to supersede his guidelines for medical behavior. The need for such a document seems great, particularly in our own times, when social evolution and revolution are extending into the areas of the provision of health care, when the immense accomplishments of research are producing moral and ethical problems of great magnitude and immediacy, when the organization and management of health services are undergoing change that is both significant and confusing, and when economic resources appear to have been stretched close to their limits in the United States, thus forcing us to set some priorities in what soon will be known as the nation's second-largest enterprise, the health business.

Especially in times such as these we are all in need of common goals and principles, a set of common denominators from which we can work, a firm platform of common purpose to which we can return for guidance, a reference standard against which we can compare our activities. If such a document is not possible, would it not be of great value to get a clearer understanding of the motivations, goals, and satisfactions of some of the world's outstanding physicians? From such a collection of personal statements the interested reader could distill aspects that have meaning for her or him. This book represents such an effort. One can hope that this collection of personal statements is a step toward a clearer definition of what physicianhood is, of that essence of doctoring that must not be tampered with as a result of our current spasms of change, lest we lose the societal space in which a profession of scientific healers can work.

Medicine has become enormously complex. Physicians these days not only carry on general patient care but may become highly trained specialists, research scientists, full-time teachers, or administrators concerning themselves with medical education, delivering health care services, or organizing our vast biomedical research efforts. A book such as this that proposes to speak of motivation must also speak to students, medical and premedical, in an effort to give them a glimpse of what it is that prompts these men and women to pursue a medical career. If this book is to have significance, the statements should be able to cross the so-called generation gap and carry an immediacy and a meaning that are, I suspect, highly personal, much the same as the Hippocratic Oath is really a very personal statement, one which affords some insight into the man Hippocrates was.

To me, the meaning of the Hippocratic Oath and the reason for its enduring value is this highly personal quality which reflects the basic concepts of devotion to people and a desire to serve them. I believe that these two concepts should be the common denominator which was mentioned earlier. In his statement, Hippocrates makes everything else emanate therefrom: the physician's relation with the patient is sacrosanct; what follows is a great respect for teaching and, by implication, for research and the acquisition of new knowledge. The humanistic basis for Hippocrates' actions is still tenable for most modern physicians and I believe for most modern medical and university students. Is it not likely that this particular interest in people is crucial not only to the makeup of the practitioner of medicine (like Hippocrates) but is also an important ingredient in the medical specialist, clinical investigator, and administrator? If so, then it is clear that school admission committees and medical educators generally should be concerning themselves more with the nature and quality of motivation in prospective medical students once a necessary basic intelligence and training level have been established. The tendency in the past fifty or sixty years has been to test motivation through the establishment of a kind of academic obstacle-survival course and to make final selections from among the survivors on the basis of academic standing. This policy has shifted somewhat in recent years, and it is hoped that the present volume will add perspectives which will enhance our consideration of this problem.

## Medical Schools

Since the early twentieth century and the Flexner Report, there has been a major emphasis in medical schools on scientific and technical competence, accomplished by setting rigorous standards and forcing students to master a certain voluminous body of knowledge. This particular characteristic of medical school, which most graduate students in the arts and sciences would find abhorrent, has not prevented an ample number of intelligent students from clamoring for entrance. At the same time, there has been an increasing amount of criticism on the part of some people regarding the dehumanization and depersonalization of medical practice. Although our whole society has undergone this same process of depersonalization, there is no simple answer to the questions raised by medical critics. Suffice it to say that the medical profession, including medical educators and our society as a whole, recognizes the great need for educating physicians motivated to deliver medical care.

I believe that medical care of the type delivered by family physicians, primary physicians, general practitioners, obstetricians, pediatricians, internists, and most surgeons must be based primarily on the desire to serve. In order to produce a growing number of people who will spend their lives in these activities, it is not enough to encourage them to read Tolstoy, Freud, and Riesman during their residency; rather, it would be ideal if they could be chosen primarily on the basis of estimating the nature of their motivation, a motivation that may have led them to concentrate in the humanities and social sciences before entering medical school.

The quality of our motivation is surely not the sole factor responsible for the dehumanizing tendencies of the twentieth century. In addition to the motivational issue, other sociologic and economic factors have played a significant role—among them the emphasis on professionalization, which occurs through long and intensely arduous training years, the excess of patient demands and expectations, and the overload of requests for help. Of interest in the latter regard is the Good Samaritan study conducted with graduating theology students at Princeton. A test situation was established for each student (unaware that he or she was participating in a test) so that he or she passed a supposed suffering fellow human being under the same conditions as did his or her colleagues, except for a number of variables: some were rushing to an appointment and some had time to spare, some thought they were on their way to give a television talk on the parable of the Good Samaritan, and others thought they were going to get an interview for a first-rate position. Reportedly, the only variable that showed a positive correlation with stopping to help the person in trouble was not being in a hurry. If this sort of thing holds true for medical practice, then it suggests that changes in the organization of health care can, in fact, be instrumental in aiding the reemergence of humanitarianism.

It seems to me that "the search for meaning" is a phrase that applies to all of us everywhere. A technocratic society such as ours, which deifies data and the hard sciences and fears platitudes, may also be a little afraid of and somewhat embarrassed by the philosophic quest for meaning. On the other hand, even our politicians recognize the nature of the problem. Listen to what Nelson Rockefeller said as long ago as 1968:

> The deepest problem before America, then, is moral or psychological. Since much of the current uneasiness reflects a search less for solutions than for meaning, remedies depend for their effectiveness on the philosophy or values which inspire them. The student unrest is impressive, not because some of it is fomented by agitators, but because it includes some of the most idealistic elements of our youth. In fact, much that disquiets us today gives us cause for hope, for it reflects not cynicism but disappointed idealism.[1]

Governor Rockefeller went on to make other observations relevant to our purposes in this book:

> Decades of "debunking" and materialism have left the young generation without moral support in face of the challenges of a revolutionary age. Leaders at all levels are seen to have been asking not too much of our people but too little. The contemporary discontent proves, among other things, that man cannot live by economics alone; he needs quality and purpose in addition to material well-being; he needs significance and meaning beyond physical comfort. The quality and success of the Peace Corps can be explained on no other ground. The spirit of idealism which it has fostered should—and can—animate our actions in meeting a wide variety of challenges.
>   For a people grown great in the experience of the frontier, the twin challenges of a technocratic bureaucracy and helping the world find a modern structure offer an adventurous opportunity. This is an exciting age. The current uneasiness exists because people care—and yet do not see the way to make their aspirations come true. The task is to prove that their aspirations are relevant and attainable. This cannot be the responsibility of the President alone; it is the responsibility of all public officials, of leaders in all walks of life—indeed, all of us.[2]

It is not difficult to list other leaders who are capable of speaking articulately about our society's goals and directions, its meaning, challenges, and opportunities. Few have spoken more poignantly about the nature and meaning of their own lives than did Dag Hammarskjöld in his autobiographical book *Markings*. Although many people may not share his religiosity, the crux of his ideas can, I believe, have significance for all of us with a major interest in medicine. Some particularly pertinent examples follow.

> Conscious of the reality of evil and the tragedy of the individual life, and conscious, too, of the demand that life be conducted with decency . . .

> To Fail—Are you satisfied because you have curbed and canalized the worst in you? In any human situation, it is cheating not to be, at every moment, one's best. How much more so in a position where others have faith in you . . .

> For someone whose job so obviously mirrors man's extraordinary possibilities and responsibilities, there is no excuse if he loses his sense of "having been called." So long as he keeps that, everything he can do has a meaning, nothing a price. Therefore: if he complains, he is accusing himself.

Finally, Hammarskjöld aims a question at his own attempts to pass wisdom on to others that he might well have aimed at all those who have written in this book:

> The scientist only records what he has been able to establish as indisputable fact. In the same way, only what is unique in a person's experience is worth writing down as a guide and a warning to others. In the same way, too, an explorer leaves it to others to pass their time taking notes on the quaint customs of the natives, or making devastating remarks about the foibles of their traveling companions.[3]

But excellence implies more than competence. It implies a striving for the highest standards in every phase of life. We need individual excellence in all forms, in every kind of creative endeavor, in political life, in education, in industry—in short, universally.[4]

The striving for excellence, the quest for meaning through service, a sense of satisfaction, and a kind of sacramental attitude concerning work are aspects of human character and personality that are not peculiar to the medical profession.[5] One would expect, in fact, that these attributes would characterize productive workers in many fields. What then, if anything, is peculiar and special about medicine?

## Different from Other Professions

It has always seemed to me that medicine as a profession offers three particular qualities to its practitioners, qualities which, indeed, do provide special benefits. The first is the constant contact with suffering and death which is afforded physicians; it is terribly difficult for sensitive physicians to ignore the realities of life, to fail to question and requestion the deeper meanings and purposes and quests of human existence, and to misappropriate their own priorities so that false values and ultimately meaningless goals become paramount. It must be admitted that there is a danger in having to face daily the human suffering and death of one's patients and friends, and that danger is a kind of fatalistic cynicism to which some doctors and nurses seem particularly prone.

The second special attribute the medical profession offers its practitioners has something to do with age—the later years of the physician's career and life. Physicians have the great opportunity of continually developing their trade. The degree to which they develop this art will, in many instances, determine their effectiveness; its development, in turn, will depend upon their continued growth as sensitive, cognitive, participating members of the human race. Thus, physicians who can maintain their scientific and technical knowledge base are offered the almost unique opportunity of becoming increasingly more valuable to and effective in society as they grow older. They seldom need to be concerned that, as they approach fifty, their job will be better done by the younger doctors. Surely, they may begin to see fewer patients, but those they see can be cared for very well. A career which offers continued, lifelong utility, with the potential for increasing value as the years go by, is a career which should be highly desirable to people seeking to live a life of high quality and excellence that is somehow related in their minds to hard work and service.

A third characteristic of medicine which makes it a special profession has to do with seeking and speaking the truth. This characteristic is at the source of the observation frequently made by outsiders when they comment on how boring it is to be with a group of doctors: "All they ever talk about is medicine!" Aside from an intrinsic interest in human biology, the ideal physician usually shares with other physicians an almost morbid concern for medical knowledge. Some newly learned fact may save an unknown patient's life; some recently published paper may indicate a way to aid in diagnosing or treating other patients whose maladies are poorly understood by the physician or whose treatment is currently unsuccessful. Sometimes physicians allow this quest for new information to become such a passion or even compulsion that they cease to develop effectively other aspects of their intellectual and aesthetic lives. Such physicians may be said to be enhancing their technical side at the expense of their "artful" side. Occasionally, of course, some physicians may develop a skill in handling various personalities far in excess of their ability to carry out the technical aspects of treating disease. At this point they may be successful and popular but perhaps inadequate. Speaking the truth has become increasingly recognized by society and profession alike as both crucial for the patient and for the trust which is the basis for the therapeutic relationship.

Medicine offers maximum opportunity for self-fulfillment, particularly for those who can either intuitively or rationally relate such fulfillment with giving of self. With every opportunity come both a responsibility and a challenge. For good physicians, the responsibility is to deliver the best possible care to their patients, and the challenge is to develop and maintain the necessary scientific and technical knowhow and personal attributes which will allow them to carry out their responsibility.

These high-sounding sentiments may have meaning for some people, but others will raise many different questions which demand answers. These days, people seem more often to question the physician's honesty and competence. Does this seriously detract from practice? What would happen if the worst fears of some people were realized and doctors became salaried? Francis Peabody said that the first role of good patient care is to care for the patient. This implies responsibility. Is the essence of the personal physician the fact that individual physicians accept personal responsibility for the health and welfare of their patients? Is that really important in practice to physicians? Must that go down the drain in the future world of supermarket medicine, where services are supplied in quantity by superb physician-technician specialists? Is there to be a role in the future for family or personal physicians and, if so, what will be their best characteristics and the nature of their work satisfactions?

What about physician-technician specialists? An objectionable term, perhaps, but more and more an appropriate one. Do we need them? Obviously! Are they an entirely different breed from the personal physician? Must they have different skills and aptitudes? Don't cardiovascular surgeons also have more than just technical responsibilities? Do they gain anything by their daily confrontation with death and long-term suffering? How can they best deal with these things—better, how can they show the rest of us how to best deal with them? Are there any rewards from caring for terminally ill patients (the threat of severe illness is, after all, usually the threat of death), and if, according to the latest style, death is only molecular disintegration, how can anyone consider it a constructive occupation to work with such patients? Does such an occupation force a special wisdom and acceptance of death on aware physicians? Are these thoughts mere platitudes?

What about medical scientists? Are they the same type of people as family physicians and physician-specialists? Do we actually divide our entering classes to medical school according to these three categories? Or should we? What are the rewards for the medical scientist or clinical investigator? Are they purely intellectual, or do action and experimentation emanate from the bedside experience? Is there a humanism here too? Or do we define clinical investigators as biologists with a primary intellectual interest in the human species?

What about clinical teachers? They used to be the practitioners who freely donated their time to passing on the art. Of late there has been a trend toward having full-time faculty members carry out most of this function. Often these people have to carry out productive research programs and seldom actually care for patients by themselves, as personal physicians must do. Does this matter? Is it good or bad? Should it be modified? What should teachers be, basically? What are their satisfactions and what is it they want to pass on to their students? Should we be teaching a method, a set of facts, a logical approach? Or should we be an example, since all the preceding things are in books, and, if an example, what sort of example?

What about medicine and society? What are medical administrators' goals, ambitions, and motivating forces? How do they get satisfaction?

> Hippocrates once said to one of his students: "Let your best means of treating people be your love for them, your interest in their affairs, your knowledge of their condition, and your recognized attentiveness to them." [6]

There is abroad an undercurrent suggesting that the solution of health manpower problems will follow hard upon the definition of the problems. Certainly our medical schools cannot produce the required number of physicians unless that number can be accurately predetermined. Perhaps by having economists define the needs in terms of the number of physicians required and by providing sufficient incentives to increase the production of physicians we will be able to produce bodies in sufficient quantity to solve the numbers and distribution problems. In fact, most recent manpower analyses conclude that the governmental programs to enhance medical school production have succeeded and that we are soon to have an excess of doctors.

I believe, however, that even if such analyses are possible they are not a true or complete solution. There may be enough doctors someday, but are there enough good doctors? Once again I would like to suggest that part of the solution lies in an understanding of motivation. If we can define what motivates happy and satisfied physicians, ones who do their job well and competently and are happy with doing it for a lifetime, ones who are capable of communicating their knowledge, advice, and concern to their patients—if we can do this, then we will be able to pick out college students with these motivations and encourage them to go to medical school. By selecting our students more on the basis of their motivations, goals, and satisfactions we will be able to produce more physicians truly concerned and vitally interested in their profession. More than the numbers will have been met; an appropriate and important step will have been taken toward resolving the problem of depersonalization.

It is my contention that there is a great untapped source of future family physicians. They are to be found among the many young men and women who never get to medical school but who have the proper motivation and basic ability to communicate with patients and who would thrive on the kinds of demands made on the practicing physician. A significant number of these students possess the necessary scientific aptitude to acquire medical skills and attain excellence in the physician's trade but too often are discouraged from medical school for invalid reasons. One of the greatest obstacles that keeps many of these people from clinical medicine could be overcome by developing a basic science aptitude test which could accurately establish at the sixteen-, seventeen-, or eighteen-year-old level whether or not the student has enough ability to succeed in medical school. The results of such a test should be made known to the students, who should then be encouraged to pursue whateve intellectual interests they wish in college, secure in the knowledge that a collegiate emphasis outside of the natural sciences will not preclude their becoming physicians and may, in fact, be helpful.

## Why This Book?

No one in my own medical student experience ever said very much that I recognized, at any rate, as dealing with some of these important matters in a meaningful way until a physician named Hermann Blumgart talked long into the night with a group of fourth-year students about caring for dying patients. Later in that same year, Chester Jones, another venerable and kind physician, in a matter of a few short minutes on two separate occasions made me feel that he was welcoming me into a very important and special profession and left me with a lasting impression of his concept of and concern for all that is involved with being a physician. It is pertinent, if somewhat distressing, to note that in my own considerable experience teaching medical students I have too seldom talked with them about this sort of thing.

Perhaps wisdom exists only in the mind of the listener or reader, but perhaps also every life incorporates or uncovers a little insight and wisdom from which others may profit. Those people who are sufficiently articulate may communicate these things. In my own life, such episodes of illumination from others occurred all too infrequently and often I did not fully understand the lasting lessons and impressions until long afterward.

In college I took an introductory course in the natural sciences given by Professor Leonard Nash. Professor Nash's lectures were intriguing partly because they were so unique. He almost never told us anything; that is, he almost never lectured. Rather, he would conduct an experiment on the stage of the lecture hall, which was just as likely not to work as it was to be successful. Only in retrospect did I realize fully that Professor Nash was setting an example for us all in his behavior and reactions, demonstrating curiosity, honesty, imagination, and persistence.

He showed us what science was by his daily interaction with it, and we learned from a master things we never forgot and could never get from a book. I am now convinced that those pedagogical lessons are among the most important and significant things I know about my own profession of teaching medical students and house officers.

After college and before medical school I spent a year at Cambridge University in England, and during this period I had an opportunity to make the acquaintance of T. S. Eliot. I had read all his works during my college years and one day spent a wonderful half hour discussing the difficulties of reconciling involvement in the affairs of people with the capacity to maintain a degree of indifference to their suffering sufficient that one would not disintegrate in the face of others' misfortunes. During the course of this animated conversation he found out that I was a Roman Catholic and later, after I had expressed some ambivalence about going to medical school, he said in a way I have never forgotten, "The world needs good Catholic doctors." Many times since I have recalled those words, which still seem to thunder down at me from some mountaintop oracle. He could just as easily have said, "The world needs good agnostic doctors" or "good atheist doctors" or "good Buddhist doctors," because what he was telling me was that the world needed good doctors and he thought I had the stuff to be one. That thought of Mr. Eliot's and his confidence in me have been very important in sustaining me through low periods in medical school and ever since.

A practicing physician once told me, when discussing his job, that some of the most rewarding experiences of his professional life came from helping and observing some of his patients as they came to terms with their own death. As he talked, I was impressed with the significance being a physician held for this man. His words and reactions evoked a response from me at a time when I was considering a medical career and his comments were, in fact, important in encouraging me to give it a try. Apparently, fewer and fewer physicians are currently transmitting similar enthusiasms to their own children, who some say are not applying to medical school to the same degree as in the past.

During my last year of medical school, a highly respected and successful practicing physician told us about the most important rule in his daily life as a physician. His rule, which he said required frequent repeating to himself, was always to sit down when visiting a patient on rounds, even if his visit was to be only thirty seconds long. He pointed out that the patient frequently relaxed, more easily communicating what was on his or her mind, or at least felt that the physician was willing to spend some time and had a personal interest in his or her patient. His obvious success in accomplishing this goal, which he demonstrated to us each day on rounds, planted seeds which are still bearing fruit.

The following statement, made in 1895 by William Osler, the father of modern American medicine, has been helpful to me again and again since the time I first came across it. It is important not only because he said it, but because so many of us can recognize the tendency to slip away from what might be considered an underlying assumption in any physician's basic philosophy.

> In these days of aggressive self assertion, when the stress of competition is so keen, and the desire to make the most of oneself so universal, it may seem a little old fashioned to preach the necessity of humility; but I insist for its own sake and for the sake of what it brings, that due humility should take the place of honour in the list. For its own sake, since with it comes not only a reverence for truth, but also a proper estimation of the difficulties encountered in our search for it. More perhaps than any other professional man, the doctor has a curious, shall I say morbid? sensitiveness to (what he regards as) personal error. In a way this is right; but it is too often accompanied by a cocksuredness of opinion, which, if encouraged, leads him to so lively a conceit that the mere suggestion of a mistake under any circumstances is regarded as a reflection of his honour, a reflection equally resented, whether of lay or professional origin. Start out with the conviction that absolute truth is hard to reach in matters relating to our fellow creatures, healthy or diseased, that slips in observation are inevitable, even with the best

trained faculties, that errors in judgement must occur in the practice of an art which consists largely in balancing possibilities—start, I say, with this in mind, and mistakes will be acknowledged and regretted; but instead of a slow process of self deception, with ever increasing inability to recognize truth, you will draw from your errors the very lessons which will enable you to avoid their repetition.[7]

We will know someday how to measure motivation, how to direct individuals with different goals and satisfactions. Right now, however, we need help from some of the more articulate and thoughtful members of our profession and its observers. This book is an attempt to get at the core of physicianhood and to approach the idea of special commitment through the articulation of a new code. The reader will find in subsequent chapters much that is highly personal and subjective on the one hand as well as objective and substantive on the other. I trust that all of it will prove either enlightening or provocative.

## Notes

1. Nelson A. Rockefeller, "Policy and the People," *Foreign Affairs* 46 (1968): 231.
2. Ibid., 234.
3. Dag Hammarskjöld, *Markings*, trans. L. Sjoberg and W. H. Auden (New York: Alfred A. Knopf, 1965), 111, 154, 156, 173.
4. J. Gardner, *Excellence: Can We Be Equal and Excellent Too?* (New York: Harper and Row, 1961), 160.
5. V. Frankl, *Man's Search for Meaning* (Boston: Beacon Press, 1962).
6. Muslim tradition.
7. William Osler, *Teacher and Student* (Philadelphia: P. Blakiston's Son and Co., 1932), 38.

# PART II.

*History, Philosophy, Ethics, Psychology, and Values Essential to Physicianhood's Core*

# 3. *Hippocrates and History: The Arrogance of Humanism*

Dickinson W. Richards

What a pleasing title this book has, and what an open invitation to any-one interested in the Father of Medicine. In this essay I shall try to accomplish several things: first, describe Hippocrates as a living person, what he looked like, how he thought and expressed himself, how he was regarded by his contemporaries of the fifth and fourth centuries B.C.; next, describe Hippocrates as a physician and surgeon, including his powers of observation and the range of his clinical experience. After this I shall consider Hippocrates' broader philosophy, his ideas about medicine and the natural order and man and nature. So much for Hippocrates himself; I shall then review the Hippocratic corpus, the whole four hundred–year collection of writings gathered under his name; then, briefly, how his views and teachings have fared down the ages; and, finally, how his ideas relate to some of the urgent problems of the present day.

Hippocrates lived during the great age of Greece. His long life (460–370 B.C.) spanned approximately those of Socrates and Plato

combined; he died when Aristotle was a young man and a decade or so
before the birth of Alexander the Great.

There are two clear references to Hippocrates by Plato, his contemporary. In the *Protagoras*[1] Socrates postulated that a young colleague, also
named Hippocrates, might go to Hippocrates of Cos, the Asklepiad, to
be instructed in medicine. (Asklepiad was a term apparently used to describe a member of the general guild of physicians.) In the *Phaedrus*[2]
Plato recorded that Hippocrates the Asklepiad teaches that an understanding of natural events is the necessary approach to a knowledge of
medicine (literally, "the body"). In his *Politics*[3] Aristotle has an interesting comment: "When one says 'the Great Hippocrates,'" he writes,
"one means not the man, but the physician." From Aristotle's brief but
authoritative statement we can deduce that Hippocrates actually lived,
he was well known to Aristotle, and a generation after his death he was
already a commanding figure. Some have even thought that there is here
an implication that Hippocrates was a man of small stature, and this
may well be so. The pertinent question is, however, what did Hippocrates indeed look like? This question has occupied archaeologists for
more than three centuries.[4]

The first evidence that was found, early in the seventeenth century,
was a Roman coin of Cos of the first century A.D., on which were depicted a head in profile, the word "hip" in Greek letters, and a serpent
staff. The head was rounded, bald, with a short beard; the nose large
with broad nares. The design is, of course, crude but gives a definite
idea of the kind of head and countenance the man had. There was much
interest through the late eighteenth and nineteenth centuries in finding
an antique sculptured head or other portrait that would resemble the
head on the coin sufficiently to enable scholars to call the head Hippocrates. There was a head in the Capitoline Museum in Rome, another of
the same man in the British Museum, and still others familiar to all and
for many years accepted as being Hippocrates. However, none of these
sculptures really fit, the faces being much narrower than that on the
coin. Half a century ago, with much additional evidence, these sculptures were clearly identified as being the Stoic philosopher Chrysippus.
There was then, at that point, no accepted representation of Hippocrates
except the coin.

In 1940, during the excavation of a burial ground near Ostia Antica,
the ancient seaport of imperial Rome, there was found within the family
tomb of a distinguished Greco-Roman physician of the first century
A.D. a pedestal on which was an inscription beginning "Life is short."
Near the pedestal on the ground was the sculptured head of an elderly
man, the right side of the face much damaged. The contour of the head
and details of the face were found to correspond closely with those on

the Roman coin of Cos. The remainder of the inscription on the pedestal did not complete the Hippocratic First Aphorism, but was an appropriate funerary sentiment: "Short is the life, but long the aeons that we mortals spend beneath the earth. To all is given part of the divine fate, whatever it be." Further examination of existing sculpture has revealed four additional heads that correspond quite closely to that at Ostia: one is in the Museo Chiaramonti, the Vatican; one in the Uffizi, Florence; one in the National Museum, Naples; and one in the Ny Carlesberg Glyptothek, Copenhagen. A fifth head, quite like the one in Copenhagen, was found thirty years ago lying in a field near Rome. All these indicated that this was a personage of note, recognized in the Greco-Roman world.

The sum total of evidence, granting that it is circumstantial, has led most archaeologists to believe with some confidence that the head represents what antiquity accepted as Hippocrates' likeness. This Ostia head is a fine Roman copy of an earlier Greek original. It is seen to be a head and countenance of great power, expressing strength and sorrow in almost equal measure, the face of a man who has seen all human experience. The Hellenistic style places the Greek original at about 280 to 300 B.C., or somewhat less than one hundred years after Hippocrates' death.

What were the enduring creations that came out of the life of this remarkable man? As in all history there are not many certainties, and we must deal with records of greatly varying authenticity.

One certainty is the Hippocratic corpus, the whole mass of medical treatises (over seventy of them still surviving) that were gathered over a period of some four hundred years and that have survived over a period of twenty-four centuries. This in itself is an astonishing product. We have, of course, writings on religion, collected over much longer periods and still with us; but where else, in either ancient or modern times, have we a collection of objective and interpretative writings, in a scientific field, assembled in one man's name over so long a period, so sedulously protected and so earnestly studied and used, over so great a span of time? Plato and Aristotle, to be sure, and of course Galen wrote more extensively, but within one or two generations they and their schools had completed their work. The Stoics continued teaching and writing for centuries, but their works were scattered, never held together by one dominating personality, and in great part lost.

It is fairly certain that there existed a school of medicine at Cos even before Hippocrates the Great.[5] His biographer, Soranus (not a reliable authority, to be sure), mentions his grandfather, Hippocrates the First, and at least two of the writings in the corpus have been dated with some assurance before Hippocrates.

What were the truly fundamental contributions to medicine of Hippocrates himself? The evidence is largely internal, and authorities naturally vary as to which treatises are "genuine," meaning by this either written by him or his immediate students or associates. I believe that by reference to a few of these one can reach the primary features of his teaching.

One of the more severe critics, Deichgraber,[6] admits only one, the *Epidemics,* Books I and III, as surely by Hippocrates himself. These are in simple form. They consist, first, of a discourse on "Constitution" (that is, the meteorological conditions and the kinds of disease occurring in a particular season) and, second, three series of detailed and exact descriptions of individual clinical cases that are, moreover, complete. These are no single visits to prestigious patients by a prestigious consultant. The physician here sees every kind of patient, from the wealthy aristocrat to the artisan, the domestic, even the slave; and he follows the patients from the beginning of the disease to its end, whether recovery or death, and whether the disease lasts two days or four months. He is concerned about the patients' mental and emotional state, as well as the physical strains or excesses that led up to the illness, and he is not in the least concerned about himself or enhancing his own reputation. Just as one example, here is a case of fulminating diphtheria:

> The woman suffering from angina (sore throat) who lay sick in the house of Aristion began her complaint with indistinctness of speech. Tongue red, and grew parched.
>
> On the first day, shivered, and grew hot.
>
> On the third day, rigor, acute fever; a reddish hard swelling in the neck, extending to the breast on either side; extremities cold and livid, breathing elevated; drink returned through the nostrils, she could not swallow, stools and urine ceased.
>
> On the fourth day, all symptoms worse.
>
> On the fifth day, she died.[7]

In the annals of medicine it would be difficult to find a more concise, exact, or vivid description of this dread disease.

This kind of exact description was new. Here is an accurate observer of natural events; not a philosopher proving a system or priest demonstrating his magic or justifying his gods. As Hippocrates himself insists over and over again, he is a practitioner of his craft, and a craft is perhaps as good a name for Hippocratic medicine as the traditional word "art," although the Greek word actually has an even larger meaning than either or both of these terms.[8]

What else does he think and do in the broad field of medicine? There are a number of other works which are considered by most authorities to have been written by Hippocrates or one of his colleagues associated in contemporary practice and teaching. The treatise *Regimen in Acute Diseases* indicates the broad principles of therapy, using the means then available: diet, purges, emetics, bleeding, and general daily regimen. The *Prognostic*[9] gives the evaluation of symptoms and signs, favorable and unfavorable. The surgical treatises on fractures, dislocations, and wounds of the head are an extraordinary group, detailing most accurately the anatomy and signs of these various injuries, when to use the knife, how to reduce the fracture or dislocation, precisely how to dress or bandage the injury, what will happen on succeeding days and how to deal with these events, right on to the long-drawn-out problems of gangrene and amputation.

Hippocrates' primary interest is in the patient and his or her care. "It is especially necessary, in my opinion," he writes, "for one who discusses this art to discuss things familiar to ordinary folk. For the subject of our inquiry is simply and solely the sufferings of these ordinary folk when they are sick or in pain."[10] His more general observations on medicine and its practice are apt to be added as terse comments in the midst of some case report or clinical discussion, like so many of our great clinicians whose finest truths are often offered, almost casually, at the bedside. "State the past, diagnose the present, foretell the future," Hippocrates wrote in the *Epidemics*. "Practise all this. As to diseases, make a habit of two things: to help, or at least not to harm. The art is of three parts: the disease, the sick man, the physician. The physician is a laborer for the art."

Here is another, from the treatise on joints (dislocations): "What you should put first in all the practise of our art is how to make the patient well; and if he can be made well in many ways, one should choose the least troublesome. This is more honorable, and more in accord with the art; that is, for anyone who is not covetous of the false coin of popular advertisement."

This discussion is most frank and outspoken. While severely criticizing unskillful practitioners, the author admits that there is much that he does not know, that he is "at a loss" about how to treat some conditions, that others will be fatal in spite of all treatment. Even more unusual, especially for that generally dogmatic philosophic age, Hippocrates is perfectly willing to describe a treatment that he has tried and that has failed. "I write this on purpose," he states, "for those things also give instruction, which after trial show themselves failures, and show why they failed." [11] Where else in ancient times can one find a natural philosopher as disarmingly honest as this? His contemporary Socrates no doubt was equally honest but hardly elsewhere in ancient times does one encounter this attitude.

This is not so much humility as it is respect, respect for human fallibility, represented here in the physician, recognition that humans cannot know all, that the best of their endeavors are limited, full of error. This is important, and I shall come back to it.

In the chapter on airs, waters, and places [12] Hippocrates reaches out further and endeavors to place humans in relation to their environment (man and nature, as it were, together): what kind of human beings develop in such and such a climate or ecological state, as well as what diseases they will have. While he describes accurately malarial climates and the chronic malarial state in humans, other sections are wide of the mark as we would interpret them now; but the point here is the breadth of Hippocrates' conception of medicine and the identification of man, both in health and disease, as a part of nature.

Hippocrates' attitude, his philosophy, at the foundation of his medical art or craft, is perhaps best set forth in a very early chapter called "Ancient Medicine." [13] In this he begins by stating that medicine has no need of hypotheses. Here one must distinguish, as Jones notes, the ancient from the modern notion of hypothesis. In the modern, a hypothesis is a postulate which, once stated, can be investigated. Not so in ancient times. Then a hypothesis was a thesis, a declaration of underlying truth, to be accepted and thereafter used to explain phenomena but never questioned. To such hypotheses Hippocrates was opposed. He does not accept, for example, Empedocles' proposition that, in order to know nature, one must first know the origin of man, how he came into being and out of what elements.

He admits certain general processes and forces, which can be derived from the study and observation of human beings. As one would expect, these are not especially original but relate to the number of philosophic generalities current in the fifth century B.C. The state of health is one of harmony, or balance of forces. [14] An acute disease, for example, with sharp acrid discharges, is caused by an imbalance of forces, to be restored by coction into thicker, more purulent secretions that lead to healing, and this through mixture or "blending." The so-called humors in this early era were recognized; they were numerous and of various kinds. The fixed doctrine came later.

In all cases the basis of medical care is to understand physis, that is, nature or the natural order. The function of medicine and the physician is to assist nature to restore the balance of forces in the body, which is the state of health.

It is necessary now to define our terms even more precisely if we are to know what Hippocrates is talking about. The word *physis* originates from a more fundamental one, meaning to grow, spring forth, or come into being. As Hippocrates uses physis, it means both the natural order in the large sense and also the nature, or constitution, of human beings. As Galdston notes, man "is in effect considered part of the natural order under whose sway he has his being." [15]

The other word of importance is *iatric,* meaning medicine or the art of healing, and this too is very broad. In Hippocrates' conception it signifies the guidance of man by the physician, in health and disease, and in all man's relations with nature. It does not include the idea of experimentation as a planned action to demonstrate a process; but Hippocrates was very much aware of the experimental or exploratory aspects of medicine. The Greek word for trial, which he uses for "treatment" in the First Aphorism,[16] shows that for him every therapeutic effort in medicine is an experiment, as indeed it is.

In this same treatise on ancient medicine, Hippocrates makes the boldest and most inclusive statement of all. "I hold," he writes, "that clear knowledge about nature can be obtained from medicine and from no other source." This is presumptuous indeed. It may be no more than a naive statement by a craftsman trying to advance the prestige of his own trade. Perhaps, but I believe that it is more than this. Since man and nature are one, we must seek this knowledge through the study of man and man in nature. This is medicine in its broadest sense. I believe that Hippocrates had this large concept in mind, though the language was not then available to give it more precise expression. There may be also the thought that at that pre-Aristotelian time, only in medicine were wholly objective observations being made.

I should mention the Hippocratic Aphorisms. These terse statements, some four hundred of them, are of variable quality and origin; many are brilliant clinical observations, many obscure and hard to interpret, many of post-Hippocratic and some of pre-Hippocratic origin. They were revered and memorized in later ages by scores of generations of Greek, Roman, Hebrew, Arabic, and medieval physicians. The First Aphorism by itself is almost a sufficient moral precept for the practice of medicine: "The life short, the art long, the right time but an instant, the trial [of therapy] precarious, the crisis grievous. It is necessary for the physician to provide not only the needed treatment, but to provide for the patient himself, and those beside him, and for his outside affairs." [17]

We must examine one more Hippocratic or early post-Hippocratic treatise, that on epilepsy—"On the Sacred Disease"—in which he contrasts medicine with religion and magic.

The name "sacred disease" for epilepsy came out of the tradition of some past age. But why this, asks Hippocrates, more than any other? All diseases are divine, he insists, and all are human. Each has a nature and proceeds according to its natural order.

Hippocrates is opposed to nonrational magic, but not at all opposed to religion in and for itself. Bring the sick man to the sanctuary, he says, "at least it is godhead that purifies and cleanses us from the greatest of our sins."

While thus not denying religion, he holds as absolutely to the mechanical order in his description of nature as Democritus himself. Incidentally, while there is multiple evidence that Hippocrates and Democritus of Abdera were friends over many years,[18] Hippocrates did not use, or appear to need, atomistic theory in all its detail. He might have been interested in Aristotle's biology, but not his cosmogony. Plato's idealism was the antithesis of Hippocrates' primary concern with objective living events. Man belongs to nature, according to Hippocrates, but nature does not belong to man. This is not a direct quotation but is, I believe, the essence of Hippocrates' attitude toward man and nature. His attitude is thus one of intense and continued inquiry into the processes of health and disease, combined with an underlying humility which recognizes his own limitations in the understanding of nature and his own fallibility in the alleviation of human suffering.

In another Mediterranean culture at about this time, the Hebrew, there were writings which proclaimed another doctrine which was to carry down through history with profound effect on future times; the doctrine that man, under a beneficent Deity, is Lord of Creation. This would appear to be the very opposite of Hippocrates' belief of man as a part of nature, as nature's servant, with nature—all knowing, all containing, and all powerful—the master. This contrast is basic to our longer story of Hippocrates and history, and we should therefore examine these Judaic writings, both in their relation to Hebrew attitudes of the time and in their later development and influence.

The particular idea of man under God as Lord of Creation is expressed most eloquently in the Old Testament:

> When I consider thy heavens, the work of thy fingers, the moon and the stars, which thou has ordained; what is man, that thou art mindful of him? and the son of man, that thou visitest him? For thou has made him a little lower than the angels, and has crowned him with glory and honour. Thou madest him to have dominion over the works of thy hands; thou has put all things under his feet;

all sheep and oxen, yea, and the beasts of the field; the fowl of the air, and the fish of the sea, and whatsoever passeth through the paths of the seas. (Psalms 8)

This seems at first sight like a broad dominion indeed, but looked at more closely one sees that the Lord has delivered to man a very limited part of nature, chiefly the living creatures with which man came in contact. All the other vast works of God are beyond man's control or understanding. In this great realm the Lord reigns and man bows down. Even within his small "dominion" man holds only a stewardship under the ever watchful eye of his Creator.

This attitude is set in its place by a consideration of the Book of Psalms as a whole. These are a collection of hymns and poems, of many ages and origins, believed now to have been assembled about the time of the building of the second temple (516 B.C.) just after the death of Cyrus the Great, or about a century before Hippocrates. There is expressed in them every kind of attitude of man toward God and God toward man:

Confidence and assurance, as in the Eighth Psalm just quoted.

Praise and adoration: "The heavens declare the glory of God; and the firmament sheweth his handiwork" (Psalms 19).

Thanksgiving and mercy: "O give thanks unto the Lord; for he is good; for his mercy endureth forever" (Psalms 136).

Trust: "I will say of the Lord, He is my refuge and my fortress; my God; in him will I trust" (Psalms 91).

Humility and fear: "For we are consumed by thine anger, and by thy wrath are we troubled. Thou hast set our iniquities before thee, our secret sins in the light of thy countenance. For all our days are passed away in thy wrath: we spend our years as a tale that is told" (Psalms 90).

Supplication: "Out of the depth have I cried unto thee, O Lord" (Psalms 130).

Despair: "My God, my God, why hast thou forsaken me?" (Psalms 22).

More profound than any of these, the Book of Job declares the all-pervading power of God and the complete and abject submission of man:

Then the Lord answered Job out of the whirlwind, and said, "Who
is this that darkeneth counsel by words without knowledge?"
". . . Where wast thou when I laid the foundations of the earth?"
[chap. 38] And he proceeds then to declare His wondrous works,
across the range of the earth, the sea, the air, and the heavens. Man
cannot comprehend the Almighty, and dares not question him. The
Lord answers Job as He answered Moses a thousand years before:
"I am that I am." [19]

With this deeper relationship between man and God (or man and nature) one can believe that Hippocrates would concur. The important later
course of the simplistic, cheerful, and confident doctrine of man as
Lord of Creation under a kindly Deity we will come back to. White
has also discussed this simplistic aspect of Judaic doctrine and its
consequences.[20]

So much for Hippocrates, the man and the physician and his teaching. Now we must pursue the adventures, misadventures, and distortions
of him and his doctrines through the course of history. We must keep
separate at all times the two main features of this teaching—one is the
actual clinical instruction in practical medicine; the other is the larger
philosophical scheme of man in nature—because these two have very
different histories.

Let us examine first the course of Hippocratic medicine within his
school itself, as more and more medical writings came to be added to
the collection. These were from many sources and with many different
philosophic backgrounds: Pythagorean, Aristotelian, Stoic, Epicurean,
and so forth. The whole, as we have it now, was probably a part of the
library of this school.

As is so often the case with a leader of thought, the wide-ranging philosophy of Hippocrates became increasingly restricted and dogmatized
as time went on, to end eventually, and unhappily, in that rigid rubric
which continued down the ages as the Hippocratic doctrine of the four
humors, combining these with the four forces or powers. This, as we
have noted, Hippocrates himself had been at much pains to denounce
as the wrong way to approach the art and science of medicine. Like so
many theories, it is so neat that it ought to be true even if it is not, and
therefore was thought worthy of being perpetuated.

Even more, perhaps, than his scientific attitude, Hippocrates as a man
was stripped of his human qualities and made into a figurehead, if not
a semideity. He was solemnly pronounced nineteenth in lineal descent
from Asklepios and twentieth in lineal descent from Hercules; he was
set up as an actual disciple of Asklepios. Nowhere is this more apparent
than in the so-called Hippocratic Oath, and one of the most refreshing

examples of recent historical criticism has been that of the late Professor Edelstein.[21] Edelstein demonstrated that the oath was not Hippocratic at all, but a sort of manifesto by a Pythagorean cult, written a generation or so after Hippocrates' death. The removal of Hippocrates from his so-called oath restores him to us as a living and responsive human being.

This is worth just a word or two of further comment. Take the oath's sententious beginning: "I swear by Apollo, physician, by Asklepios, by Hygeia, by Panacea, by all the gods and goddesses," and so forth and so forth. In the true Hippocratic writings, Hippocrates does not swear, either by Apollo or anyone else. Least of all would he have sworn by Asklepios and the latter's supposititious daughters, Hygeia and Panacea. Hippocrates' doctrine of rational medicine was the opposite of the Asklepian rites of magic and dream-ritual, for which he had nothing but contempt. In the genuine Hippocratic writings the name of Asklepios is never even mentioned. There is, in fact, a legend cited by Pliny that Hippocrates himself burned to the ground an earlier temple of Asklepios on the Island of Cos.[22] Though probably apocryphal, this legend may still represent Hippocrates' opinion. Similarly, all the strong provisions in the oath against surgery, therapeutic abortion, and so forth are wholly in accord with Pythagorean doctrine and wholly at variance with the Hippocratic doctrine. Thus, the so-called Hippocratic Oath is not Hippocratic but a document written a generation after Hippocrates died by another later cult of philosophers and physicians.

Upon reflection, is it not odd that for thousands of years hundreds of thousands of eager young physicians should have employed the first moment of their medical careers in swearing a mighty oath, whereas the Father of Medicine himself never saw the oath, never swore this oath, and indeed, so far as the record goes, never swore at all? There are, of course, many excellent ethical precepts in the oath; these also can be found, stated in brief and reasonable words, in the true writings of Hippocrates.

In the later works of the corpus, if one leaves aside the medical philosophy and looks only at the medical and surgical observation, one finds that there still is much of value and of the widest range. This solid foundation of practical clinical medicine is what continued to be valued by successive generations of physicians, and what therefore held the corpus together as a sort of textbook on a grand scale. The long list of commentators provides abundant proof of this. Aristotle comments on the treatise "The Nature of Man"; his student, Menon, lists a number of the writings.[23] Herophilus, the anatomist of the Alexandrian school around 300 B.C., was a commentator, and so, more extensively, was his student Bacchius. Eoritan, in the time of Nero, listed the works known to him. To complete our study, the great Renaissance compiler and editor, Anutius Foesius, assembled some two hundred commentators—Greek, Roman, Hebrew, and Arabic, as well as medieval and Renaissance—on the works of Hippocrates.[24]

But it was, of course, Galen at the end of the second century A.D. who truly and authoritatively brought to life again the major writings of the Hippocratic school. It is extraordinary how absolute was the devotion this arrogant and overweening man paid to the Father of Medicine. To be sure, if Galen did not agree with the Hippocratic writing, he sometimes reinterpreted it in the direction of his own ideas. He wrote commentaries on or mentioned over thirty chapters, including all but one of those that we now accept as "genuinely" Hippocratic.[25] It is interesting that Galen does not mention the oath. But Galen also accepted, and made his own, that same rigid humoral philosophy worked out in the post-Hippocratic period, and he successfully passed this on to later Roman and medieval times.

We can skip now over vast centuries. With medical theory and philosophy fixed and with experimental inquiry as yet unborn, practical medical knowledge was derived largely from the ancients, and even this in fragmentary form. Some of Galen's medicine and physiology survived; much is of his materia medica. Greek medicine was delivered largely through Arabic sources, though Hippocrates' *Aphorisms, Prognostic,* and *Dietetics* were available in Latin translation.

These sources formed the textbooks in the better schools for a thousand years. Surgery declined to the level of barber-surgeon practitioners. Medicine as a practical healing art was reduced to bleeding, purging, and using empirical formulae mixed with astrology, superstition, and magic. Its total impotence during the ravages of the Black Death, from the mid-fourteenth century on, diminished its standing still further.

Medicine was late in joining the Revival of Learning, slumbering on in Galenic tradition for nearly two centuries after the first flowering of art and literature in Italy. This was only partly because of the stubborn adherence of medical leaders to Galenic doctrine, partly because other science was late in starting, and partly also because the full texts of the medical knowledge of the ancients arrived from the East only toward the end of the fifteenth and early sixteenth centuries. The Hippocratic corpus was a part of this new or newly restored learning. The first editions of the corpus, with Latin translations, were published in 1525 and 1526.

This was a time of great events, in which, as it turned out, Hippocrates and his doctrines played a diminishing role. Let us consider again the two aspects of this doctrine: on the one hand, the clinical descriptions and teaching, and on the other, the broader ideas of medicine and philosophy. In the former, as one would expect, it was the clinicians

who avidly seized upon the newly discovered writings, whereas the ana-
tomists and physiologists, such as Vesalius and William Harvey, stayed
with Galen and Aristotle, at least as long as they could.

Outstanding among these clinicals were Ambroise Paré of France in
the sixteenth century, Thomas Sydenham of England in the seventeenth
century, and Hermann Boerhaave of Holland in the early eighteenth century. Paré, the surgeon, contemporary of Vesalius, was a man of humble
origin and no learning. It has been thought that he hired some assistant
to put into his writings Hippocratic quotations, but Paré did more than
this. In his great textbook of surgery, the section on fractures and dislocations is modelled exactly after the Hippocratic treatises; in fact, it
reads like an extension of these.[26] Paré was a true disciple of the Father
of Medicine. Thomas Sydenham went further: not only did he follow, in
his textbook *Processus Integri,* the Hippocratic method of exact clinical
description, but he accepted also his broader ideas of health and disease
in the natural order and made explorations in the field of epidemiology.
These, however, were not taken up by his successors and were soon
forgotten.

But these more or less isolated events in clinical medicine, over a
two-century span, are small indeed when compared to the momentous
discoveries and revolutions in the whole realm of science. I realize that
these are familiar to everyone, but I must look at them briefly in their
relation to medicine, both looking backward to the ancients and forward
as they transformed all science, philosophy, and society in the generations ahead. The dominant force, of course, was the discovery and
elaboration of the methods of experiment, which had been absent from
the work of almost all in ancient times.

There was a resurrection also of the old Judaic, now Judeo-Christian,
doctrine of man as Lord of Creation under a beneficent Deity. This belief, which we left with the Hebrews two thousand years back, had had
a variable course down the centuries. There had been a reappearance
with the "good news" of earlier Christianity, and from then on it was
strengthened in good times when God was merciful and man prospered,
blotted out in times of poverty, defeat, pestilence, and despair, or when
some priest or prophet thundered God's wrath and damnation, and even
Christ was preached more as judge than as savior.

But in the late sixteenth century and throughout the seventeenth century (the "Century of Genius") the exhilaration of discovery pervaded
all Western Europe, especially as freedom of thought finally emerged
from the repression of the Church. Yet most of the great scientists of the
age—one thinks especially of the British school, Robert Boyle, Isaac
Newton, Stephen Hales—were devout and pious men who recognized in
all humility the limitations of their work and set forth their discoveries

as demonstrations of the wondrous works of God.[27] Just as with the early Hebrews, theirs was not only an inquiry but a stewardship under the surveillance of an all-wise Creator, and in no sense a conquest.

In the eighteenth century the scene changed again. This was the Age of Enlightenment, in philosophy, literature, science, and politics. Disregarding Voltaire's satire, the general view was that indeed "all was for the best, in the best of all possible worlds."

In the physical sciences in this brave new world man was all but overwhelmed by his own success. Whitehead has said that "the Middle Ages were the Age of Faith based on Reason, the eighteenth century the Age of Reason based on Faith."[28] It was faith in science and its limitless possibilities. It was also faith in man and his limitless capability. The Deity was referred to as Divine Providence and appeared to be benign and in accord with man as prospective Lord of Creation. The earlier doctrine of Francis Bacon, that knowledge is power, gave philosophic blessing to the advances of technology. Man was the master; nature in its limitless profusion was his servant. There was something also of the crusader added to the conception: man conquering the infidels of a baleful nature, or at least the baleful and antihuman features of man's environment. In any event, the prospect was pleasing. By taking thought and exerting himself, man would soon learn to live forever in prosperity and peace. The immense achievements of science and technology through the eighteenth and nineteenth centuries could not but serve as proof of the validity of this conception. By the end of the nineteenth century Providence disappeared, man was on his own, and the Age of Humanism had arrived.

In the new scheme of things it is apparent that Hippocrates' ideas had long faded into the background. As emphasized recently by Galdston, whatever was left of the Hippocratic idea of medicine assisting nature in the restoration of health gave way to the experimental approach and its consequences.[29] Diseases became specific entities with etiologic agents, cures, and preventions, and in the ever-strengthening anthropocentric philosophy of our age they came to be looked upon as enemies to be put down and stamped out under the foot of the Lord of Creation. Each discovery was another battle won in man's total conquest of nature. One by one, infections, surgical conditions, deficiency states, and metabolic defects have been brought under control by surgery, miracle drugs, or other agents; even persisting chronic diseases have been alleviated. In our environment, pests unfavorable to our food products, either animal or vegetable, have been destroyed by powerful poisons and predatory animals wiped out. Heredity in plants and animals has been rearranged to benefit humans and even in humans, heredity is about to be placed under favorable control, at least in the minds of some. Man has, in fact, all but reached his goal as Lord of Creation. Even two world wars, with their insane and ghastly devastation, did not disturb the dream, still resting in the confident scientific philosophy of the eighteenth century.

Then, at first slowly, later with increasing momentum, something happened. God disappeared from his heaven, and all was not right with the world. Man's power became ever greater, but this, curiously, made matters worse and not better, because his power became too great for his own understanding and moved even further beyond his awareness of consequences. It began to be apparent that on this earth there is no longer a physical frontier: the limitless horizons of the eighteenth century have been closed in. One physical event, man-induced, can reach around the world. There is now no place to hide, as many have said on numerous occasions.

One is reminded of that moment in the life of Niels Bohr,[30] that great and good man, when he awoke to the somber realization that the true and the good are not the same, that the true, in fact, can be appallingly evil. I refer, obviously, to the explosion of the first atomic bomb. There is no need to continue this story: everyone is aware of the subsequent destruction, the radioactivity that has been loosed upon the world, and the present threat of annihilation. It was the same event that brought Robert Oppenheimer to remark, drily, that for the first time science has discovered the meaning of sin.

But already man, in his rash expenditure of power, has pushed nature beyond its capacity. Nature is no longer indefinitely extensive and extending; it is returning upon itself, and upon us. Man's unbridled use of his technological armament throws whole segments of the natural order out of balance, with the full meaning of this obscure, the outcome unknown.

In a word, the world has moved from an open to a closed system. This is something new for the world, or at least newly apprehended, and it must be reckoned with, because it is irrevocable. Examples of this are everywhere and beyond enumeration, but a few may be identified.

Having reached this point, this crisis or turning point in the world's history, we must (as my further argument) consider how it relates to our prime dilemma: the established and still believed eighteenth-century philosophy versus that of our now forgotten friend Hippocrates. Is man still master of his fate, still Lord of Creation, and, if not, what are his prospects?

There are two worlds: the world of nature and the world of man; or, if you prefer, the ecological world and the politico-socio-military-economic world, each acting on the other. I appreciate that everyone these days is talking, writing, meeting, protesting, and organizing on all these problems; any repetition would seem unnecessary. But perhaps I can identify a very few and then suggest how Hippocrates might respond to the situation before us, which, after all, is the topic I began with.

However much we don't like to talk or even think about it these days, the nuclear sword of Damocles hangs over us all the same, the sword heavier with each succeeding year and the thread more tenuous. We do not even know what our existing excess radiation will have done a century from now. And the politico-military industrialists go on building up, and building, the supplies above and beneath the earth and placing them in trigger-releasable form, at least in Russia and the U.S.A. Small bits of information about these materials filter through the politico-military curtain from time to time.

There is that curious Pentagonian euphemism called Broken Arrow, "accidental damage to a nuclear weapon, resulting in actual or potential hazard to life and property." [31] There have been several of these, from crash of bombers and breakage of hydrogen bombs, releasing plutonium dust. I know very little about these things, but read that this radioactive substance has a half-life of 24,000 years, and two-billionths of a gram is lethal to a human being. One such event occurred in northern Spain in 1966, turning the area into a radioactive wasteland; another in northern Greenland in 1968, causing the military to spend millions frantically digging and dredging up tons of radioactive snow and ice.

Then there is the Hanford Atom Products Operation in south-central Washington State, where in the years just before and after the end of World War II the Hanford reactors produced, in the words of Sheldon Novick, "enough plutonium to end the world in one incandescent flash." [32] Now there are stored there, in addition, in steel and concrete tanks seventy-five million gallons of intensely active radioactive wastes, "about as much radioactivity as would be produced by the explosion of all the plutonium war heads in our nuclear stockpile." It was not realized at the time these were built that this is a fairly active earthquake area, and the tanks were not built to withstand such shocks. Dr. Glenn T. Seaborg of the Atomic Energy Commission, commenting at the end of Novick's paper, while not denying the inadequacy of early geologic surveys, states that all this has been checked and the Atomic Energy Commission is watching the situation and working to solidify the wastes. We hope so. The main point here, however, is the magnitude of even the secondary possibilities of our nuclear threat. We applaud the peaceful uses of nuclear power, but what are the consequences of the heat and other effluents into nearby waters, and of possible diffusion of radioactive tritium into the air? [33]

Here is another problem that we do talk about. DDT was hailed as a great discovery, and indeed it was. Who would have thought it would persist and find its way into fish and bird life, to the extinction by sterilization of countless millions? It also is in us. What will it do to us? We don't exactly know. There are, of course, strong and probably eventually effective measures to eliminate DDT. But are other pesticides any better?

The Canadian government, more forthright than some others in such matters, distributes information on the present state of affairs; for example, in the fruit-growing regions milder pesticides which soon lose their effectiveness are being succeeded by stronger chemicals.[34] What do we know about the late or ultimate effects of these chemicals? The farm hands, formerly spraying in blue denims, now have to wear insulating suits and masks. But they are in a bind: the pestiferous insects are still becoming immune and increase, while the favorable predatory insects have all been killed off and the birds and insect-eating animals killed or driven away.[35] Yet if the farmers do not spray they lose 30 percent of their crop sales. And who can stand up against the power of money?

Take oil and the other fossilized fuels that have so fabulously enriched so many and brought prosperity and material benefits to untold thousands across the world. The primary product of combustion, carbon dioxide, while colossal, seems now likely to be controllable, at least for a while, because of the vast absorbing capacity of our oceans, so that the "hothouse effect" will not be death-dealing.[36] Of course, there is prodigious pollution by other gases within populated places, but these are small compared with the world's surface and are receiving much attention anyway.

What about the never-ending spillage and outpouring of oil and its various products of combustion down our streams into coastal waters and out on the open ocean, destroying uncountable quantities of aquatic and marine life of all varieties and in all stages of their life cycles?[37] When Thor Heyerdahl reports the same fouling of surface water all across the Atlantic, we can wonder what other poisons such as DDT are doing to the surface and life below.[38] We know, incidentally, that it is marine plant life which is largely responsible for the replenishment of atmospheric oxygen (though the cycle is a slow one).[39] Is this not cause for some concern? Politicians make high-sounding speeches about how all this will be brought under strict control; but the dire demand now in economic terms is simply that almost everything moves by oil and the larger part of all our applied energy is supplied by this substance. Knowing this we are forced to ask, will there ever be control, or can there be?

Other local ravages of waters, forests, and minerals by many industries and many governments are being more seriously dealt with, because humans with their myopic vision can discern them. But still the wastage goes on.

Population, of course, presents another vast problem. Solutions are technically feasible but socially generations away. It has not reached a point of disaster in this country but it has in India, and other crowded nations are not far from it.

And then there is war, even more costly and dehumanizing at home as power increases; devastating, ghastly, and genocidal abroad. But war on this scale seems now to be strictly an American specialty, and I should apologize to Hippocrates for being so parochial. However, he would understand. He was said to have been an honorary citizen of Athens, and he saw the greatness, the defeat, and the downfall of Athens and lived for a score of years after. (This reputed honor was probably apocryphal, but then so is my scenario.) In the prosperous days of Athens one imagines how he might have called on one of his comfortable Athenian patients sitting in his olive grove with his friends and heard them say of their enemies, by Zeus, after all, why do we bother, why not just go over and kill them all?

Finally, we return to our primary question: how about man as Lord of Creation? If one is to be Lord of Creation, one must foresee all, anticipate all consequences, not wait for disaster to occur (unknown or even unimagined), then frantically spend half one's time and energy correcting past blunders. But man does not anticipate and he does not or has not the knowledge to count the costs. If one is to be Lord of Creation one must act for the good of all, not for a favored few. Man acts for the favored few, the strong against the weak.

The plain fact is, man is not Lord of Creation and never will be. Once an eager explorer, then a confident builder, he has become, by a curious turn of fate, the destroyer, at the moment destroying his habitation and not far from destroying himself. "They have sown to the wind," said the prophet three centuries before Hippocrates, "and they shall reap the whirlwind" (Hosea 8:7).

And nature, on her side, can indeed be deranged, but if sufficiently deranged could she not simply dispose of her one-time little conqueror?

> Man, proud man
> Drest in a little brief authority,
> Most ignorant of what he's most assured,
> His glassy essence, like an angry ape,
> Plays such fantastic tricks before high heaven
> As make the angels weep. (Shakespeare, *Measure for Measure*)

Or if you find Shakespeare bitter, try Euripides:

> Oh, vain is man,
> Who glorieth in his joy, and hath no fears,

> While to and fro the chances of the years
> Dance like an idiot in the wind. (Euripides, *Daughters of Troy*)

It is not hard to judge how Hippocrates would react to all this; how he would accept, in our present circumstances, the somber verdict of the two tremendous visionaries whom I have just quoted, one of them an immediate contemporary, the other flourishing two thousand years after. Hippocrates would stress that man must be the servant of nature and can never be its master; man must be nature's protector, and not its despoiler; nature is now seen to be finite and limited, yet man is more finite and infinitely more limited. Man must have respect, as Hippocrates himself did, for his own errors and frailties. With the "chances of the years," by reason of man's immense and ill-expended power, the world has reached a turning point: it is now a closed system. Man has himself now passed his day of freedom on this planet; he cannot have all he wants, but he must learn what things are too big for him—too big for his conquest, too big for his consciousness.[40] In the larger humanism, man must learn to conform, not imperiously strive to impose his will on things infinitely greater and more complex than he is.

All this is easy to say, hard to do. There must be a program, no doubt. What I am arguing for is not a program—I have none—but a state of mind. The Lord and nature know and are in ultimate command; man does not know and is not in command. He needs vast extension of his knowledge—everyone is aware of this. His search into the unknown will always be incomplete and inadequate—everyone is not aware of this. If the Lord and nature are ruthless at times, they keep the world in balance. If man is even to approach this, he needs more than knowledge, he must have responsibility, humility, magnanimity, self-denial—in science, government, industry, education, by all those in power everywhere.

Can man measure up, and is there still time? Who can tell?

These are some of the considerations that emerge from a contemplation of Hippocrates and history.

# Notes

1. Plato, *Protagoras*, 311, B.
2. Plato, *Phaedrus*, 270, C–E.
3. Aristotle, *Politics*, VII 4, 1326a.
4. G. M. A. Richter, *Portraits of the Greeks* (London: Phaidon Press, 1965).
5. W. H. S. Jones, *Hippocrates I*, Loeb Classical Library (London: William Heinemann, 1923).
6. K. Deichgraber, "Die Epidemien und das Corpus hippokraticum," *Abhandlungen der preussischen Akad der Wissenschaften: Phil-hist Klasse* 3 (1933).
7. Hippocrates, Epidemics III, Case VII, in Jones, *Hippocrates I*.

8. D. W. Richards, "Medical Priesthoods, Past and Present," in *Transactions of the Association of American Physicians* (Baltimore, 1962).

9. W. H. S. Jones, *Hippocrates II,* Loeb Classical Library (London: William Heinemann, 1923).

10. Jones, *Hippocrates I.*

11. E. T. Withington, *Hippocrates III,* Loeb Classical Library (London: William Heinemann, 1928).

12. Jones, *Hippocrates I.*

13. Ibid.

14. Ibid.

15. I. Galdston, "The Decline and Resurgence of Hippocratic Medicine," *Bulletin of the New York Academy of Medicine* 44 (1968): 1237.

16. D. W. Richards, "The First Aphorism of Hippocrates," *Perspectives in Biology and Medicine* 5 (1961): 61.

17. Ibid.

18. Diogenes Laertius, *Lives of the Philosophers,* Bohn's Classical Library (London, 1853).

19. R. B. Chamberlin and H. Feldman, *The Dartmouth Bible* (New York: Houghton Mifflin, 1965).

20. L. White, Jr., "The Historical Roots of Our Ecological Crisis," *Science* 155 (1967): 203–207.

21. L. Edelstein, "The Hippocratic Oath: Text, Translation and Interpretation," *Bulletin of the History of Medicine,* suppl. 1 (1943).

22. A. Herzog, *Kos Asklepieion,* vol. 1 of *Ergebnissen der deutschen Ausgrabungen und Forschungen* (Berlin: Heinrich Keller, 1932).

23. Jones, *Hippocrates I.*

24. A. Foesius, *Magni Hippocratis medicorum omnium facile princeps, opera omnia quae extant* (Geneva: Samuel Chouet, 1657).

25. F. H. Garrison, *An Introduction to the History of Medicine* (Philadelphia: W. B. Saunders, 1924).

26. D. W. Richards, "Shock and Collapse in Internal Medicine," in *VII International Congress of Internal Medicine* (Stuttgart: Georg Thieme, 1963).

27. S. Hales, *Vegetable Staticks* (1727).

28. A. N. Whitehead, *Science and the Modern World* (New York: Macmillan, 1925).

29. Galdston, "Decline and Resurgence."

30. R. Moore, *Niels Bohr, His Science, and the World They Changed* (New York: Alfred A. Knopf, 1966).

31. J. Larus, "Nuclear Accidents and the ABM," *Saturday Review,* May 31, 1969.

32. S. Novick, "Earthquake at Gaza," *Environment* 12 (January 1970).

33. E. P. Radford et al., "Nuclear Power Plants of the Chesapeake Bay: A Statement of Concern," *Environment* 11 (September 1969).

34. Canadian Government Department of Agriculture, documentary film, 1969.

35. J. C. Dickinson III, "Hydra-headed Pesticides," *Science* 171 (1971): 16.

36. President's Science Advisory Committee, Office of Science and Technology, "Restoring the Quality of Our Environment," in *Report of the Environmental Panel* (Washington, D.C., November 1965).

37. P. H. Abelson, "Marine Pollution," *Science* 171 (1971): 21.

38. T. Heyerdahl, *National Geographic Magazine* (January 1971): 55.

39. President's Science Advisory Committee, "Restoring the Quality."

40. I. Galdston, "Prometheus and the Gods: An Essay on Ecology," *Bulletin of the New York Academy of Medicine* 40 (1964): 560.

# 4. *Toward an Expanded Medical Ethics: The Hippocratic Ethic Revisited*

Edmund D. Pellegrino

Good physicians are by the nature of their vocation called upon to practice their art within a framework of high moral sensitivity. For two millennia this sensitivity was provided by the oath and the other ethical writings of the Hippocratic corpus. No code has been more influential in heightening the moral reflexes of ordinary individuals. Every subsequent medical code is essentially a footnote to the Hippocratic precepts, which even to this day remain the paradigm of how good physicians should behave.

The Hippocratic ethic is marked by a unique combination of humanistic concern and practical wisdom admirably suited to physicians' tasks in society. In a simpler world, that ethic long sufficed to guide physicians in their service to patient and community. Today, the intersections of medicine with contemporary science, technology, social organization, and changed human values have revealed significant missing dimensions in the ancient ethic. The reverence we rightly accord the Hippocratic precepts must not obscure the need for a critical examination of their missing dimensions—those most pertinent for contemporary physicians and society. The need for expanding traditional medical ethics is already well established. It was first underscored by the shocking revelations of the Nuremberg trials.

A spate of new codes has appeared which attempt to deal more responsibly with the promise and the dangers of human experimentation; the inquiry is well under way.[1] More recently, further ethical inquiries have been initiated to reflect the change in moral climate and medical attitudes toward abortion, population control, euthanasia, transplanting organs, and manipulating human behavior and genetic constitution.[2] In actual fact, some of the major proscriptions of the Hippocratic Oath are already being consciously compromised: confidentiality can be violated under certain conditions of law and public safety, abortion is being legalized, dangerous drugs are used everywhere, and a conscious but controlled invasion of the patient's rights in human experimentation is now permitted.

This essay will examine some important dimensions of medical ethics not included in the Hippocratic ethic and, in some ways, even obscured by its too rigorous application. To be considered here are the ethics of participation, the questions raised by institutionalizing medical care, the need for an axiology of medical ethics, the changing ethics of competence, and the tensions between individual and social ethics.

An analysis of these questions will reveal the urgent need for expanding medical ethical concerns far beyond those traditionally observed. A deeper ethic of social and corporate responsibility is needed to guide the profession to levels of moral sensitivity more congruent with the expanded duties of the physician in contemporary culture.

The normative principles which constitute what may loosely be termed the Hippocratic ethic are contained in the oath and the deontological books: *Law, Decorum, Precepts,* and *The Physician.* These treatises are of varied origin and combine behavioral imperatives derived from a variety of sources—the schools at Cos and Cnidus intermingled with Pythagorean, Epicurean, and Stoic influences.[3]

The oath speaks of the relationships of the student and his teacher, advises the physician never to harm the patient, enjoins confidentiality, and proscribes abortion, euthanasia, and the use of the knife.[4] It forbids sexual commerce with the women in the household of the sick. The doctor is a member of a select brotherhood dedicated to the care of the sick, and his major reward is a good reputation.

*Law* discusses the qualities of mind and the diligence required of the prospective physician from early life. *The Physician* emphasizes the need for dignified comportment, a healthy body, a grave and kind mien, and a regular life. In *Decorum,* we are shown the unique practical wisdom rooted in experience which is essential to good medicine and absent in the quack; proper comportment in the sick room dictates a reserved, authoritative, composed air; much practical advice is given on the arts and techniques of clinical medicine.[5] *Precepts* again warns against theorizing without fact, inveighs against quackery, urges consideration in setting fees, and encourages consultation in difficult cases.[6]

Similar admonitions can be found scattered throughout the Hippocratic corpus, but it is these few brief ethical treatises which have formed the character of the physician for so many centuries. From them, we can extract what can loosely be called the Hippocratic ethic—a mixture of high ideals, common sense, and practical wisdom. A few principles of genuine ethics are often repeated and intermingled with etiquette and homespun advice of all sorts. The good physician emerges as an authoritative and competent practitioner devoted to his patient's well-being. He is a benevolent and sole arbiter who knows what is best for the patient and makes all decisions for him.

There is in the Hippocratic corpus little explicit reference to the responsibilities of medicine as a corporate entity with responsibility for its members and duties to the greater human community. The ethic of the profession as a whole is assured largely by the moral behavior of its individual members. There is no explicit delineation of the corporate responsibility of physicians for one another's ethical behavior. On the whole, the need for maintaining competence is indirectly stated. There are, in short, few explicit recommendations about what we would today call "social ethics."

These characteristics of the Hippocratic ethic have been carried forward to our day. They are extended in the code of Thomas Percival which formed the basis of the first code of ethics adopted by the American Medical Association in 1847.[7] They were sufficient for the less complex societies of the ancient and modern worlds but not for the contemporary twentieth-century experience. The Hippocratic norms can no longer be regarded as unchanging absolutes but as partial statements of ideals in need of constant reevaluation, amplification, and evolution.

Without in any way denigrating the essential worth of the Hippocratic ethic, it is increasingly apparent that the ideas conveyed about the physician are simplistic and incomplete for today's needs. In some ways, it is even antipathetic to the social and political spirit of our times. For example, the notion of the physician as a benevolent and paternalistic figure who decides all for the patient is inconsistent with today's educated public. It is surely incongruous in a democratic society in which the rights of self-determination are being assured by law. In a day when the remote effects of individual medical acts are so consequential, we cannot be satisfied with an ethic which is so inexplicit about social responsibilities. Nowhere in the Hippocratic Oath is the physician recognized as a member of a corporate entity which can accomplish good ends for humanity that are more than the sum of individual good acts. The necessity for a stringent ethic of competence and a new ethic of shared responsibility which flows from team and institutional medical care is understandably not addressed.

It is useful to examine some of these missing ethical dimensions as examples of the kind of organic development long overdue in professional medical ethical codes.

The central and most admirable feature of the oath is the respect it inculcates for the patient. In the oath, the doctor is pledged always to help patients and keep them from harm. This duty is then exemplified by specific prohibitions against abortion, use of deadly drugs, surgery, breaches of confidence, and indulgence in sexual relations with members of the sick person's household. Elsewhere, in *The Physician, Decorum,* and *Precepts,* the physician is further enjoined to be humble, careful in observation, calm and sober in thought and speech. These admonitions have the same validity today that they had centuries ago and are still much in need of cultivation.

But in one of these same works, *Decorum,* we find an excellent example of how drastically the relationship between physician and patient has changed since Hippocrates' time. The doctor is advised to "Perform all things calmly and adroitly, concealing most things from the patient while you are attending him." A little further on, the physician is told to treat the patient with solicitude, "revealing nothing of the patient's present and future condition."[8] This advice is at variance with social and political trends and with the desires of most educated patients. It is still too often the modus operandi of physicians dreaming of a simpler world in which authority and paternalistic benevolence were the order of the day.

Indeed, a major criticism of physicians today centers on this very question of disclosure of essential information. Many educated patients feel frustrated in their desire to participate in decisions which affect them as intimately as medical decisions invariably do. The matter really turns on establishing new bases for the patient's trust. The knowledgeable patient can trust the physician only if he or she feels the latter is competent and uses that competence with integrity and for ends which have value for the patient. Today's educated patient wants to understand what the physician is doing, why he or she is doing it, what the alternatives may be, and what choices are open. In a democratic society, people expect the widest protection of their rights to self-determination.

Hence, contemporary patients have a right to know the decisions involved in managing their cases.

When treatment is specific, with few choices open, the prognosis good, the side effects minimal, disclosing the essential information is an easy matter. Unfortunately, medicine frequently deals with indefinite diagnoses and nonspecific treatments of uncertain value. Several alternatives are usually open; prognosis may not be altered by treatment; side effects are often considerable and discomfort significant. The patient certainly has the right to know these data before therapeutic interventions are initiated. The Nuremberg code and others were designed to protect the subject in the course of human experimentation by insisting on the right of informed and free consent. The same right should be guaranteed in the course of ordinary medical treatment as well.

So fundamental is this right of self-determination in a democratic society that to limit it, even in ordinary medical transactions, is to propagate an injustice. This is not to ignore the usual objections to disclosure: the fear of inducing anxiety in the patient, the inability of the sick patient to participate in the decision, the technical nature of medical knowledge, and the possibility of litigation. These objections deserve serious consideration but will, on close analysis, not justify concealment except under special circumstances. Obviously, the fear of indiscriminate disclosure cannot obfuscate the invasion of a right, even when concealment is in the interest of the patient.

Surely physicians are expected by patients and society to use disclosure prudently. For the very ill, the very anxious, the poorly educated, the too young, or the very old, doctors will permit themselves varying degrees of disclosure. The modes of doing so must be adapted to the patient's educational level, psychological responses, and physiologic state. It must be emphatically stated that the purpose of disclosure of alternatives, costs, and benefits in medical diagnosis and treatment is not to relieve the physician of the onus of decision or displace it on the patient. Rather, it permits the physician to function as technical expert and adviser, inviting the patient's participation and understanding as aids in the acceptance of the decision and its consequences. This is the only basis for a mature, just, and understandable physician-patient relationship.

The most important human reason for enabling patients to participate in the decisions which affect them is to allow consideration of their personal values. Here, the Hippocratic tradition is explicitly lacking, since its spirit is almost wholly deontological; that is, obligations are stated as absolutes without reference to any theory of values. Underlying value systems are not stated or discussed. The need for examining the intersection of values inherent in every medical transaction is unrecognized. The values of the physician or of medicine are assumed to prevail as absolutes, and an operational attitude of noblesse oblige is encouraged.

A deontologic ethic was not inappropriate for Greek medicine, which did not have to face so many complex and antithetical courses of action. But a relevant ethic for our times must be more axiologic than deontologic; that is, based on a more conscious theory of values. The values upon which any action is based are of enormous personal and social consequence. An analysis of conflicting values underlies the choice of a noxious treatment for a chronic illness, the question of prolonging life in an incurable disease, or setting priorities for using limited medical resources. Instead of absolute values, we deal more frequently with an intersection of several sets and subsets of values: those of the patient, the physician, sciences, and society. Which shall prevail when these values are in conflict? How do we decide?

The patient's values must be respected whenever possible and whenever they do not create injustice for others. Patients are free to delegate the decision to their physicians, but they must do this consciously and freely. To the extent that they are educated, responsible, and thoughtful, modern individuals will increasingly want the opportunity to examine relative values in each transaction. When patients are unconscious or otherwise unable to participate, the physician or the family acts as their surrogate, charged as closely as possible to preserve their values.

The Hippocratic principle of *primum non nocere,* therefore, must be expanded to encompass the patient's value system if it is to have genuine meaning. To impose the doctor's value system is an intrusion on the patient; it may be harmful, unethical, and result in an error in diagnosis and treatment. Further, the concept of "health" as a positive entity is as vague today as in Hippocrates' time. Its definition is highly personal. The physician's view of health may be quite at variance with that of the patient or even of society. Doctors understandably tend to place an ideological value on health and medicine. Society should expect this from them as experts, but their views must not prevail unchallenged. Indeed, society must set its own priorities for health. The amelioration of social disorders like alcoholism, sociopathy, drug addiction, and violence can have greater value for a healthy human existence, for example, than merely prolonging life in patients with chronic disabling disorders. Indeed, the patient and society now demand to participate in making the choices. The configuration of value choices each of us makes defines concretely our uniqueness and individuality. Hence, each patient has a slightly different definition of health. Physicians are also individuals with sets of values which invariably color their professional acts. Their views of sex, alcohol, suffering, poverty, race, and so forth can sharply differ with those of their patients. Their advice on these matters, as well as their definition of cooperation, often has a strong ideologic or moralistic tinge. Physicians must constantly guard against confusing their own values as the "good" to which all must subscribe if they desire to be treated by them.

Disclosure is, therefore, a necessary condition if we really respect each patient as a unique being whose values, as a part of his or her person, are no more to be violated than his or her body. The deontologic thrust of traditional medical ethics is too restrictive in a time when the reexamination of all values is universal. It even defeats the very purposes of the traditional ethic, which are to preserve the integrity of the patient as a person.

Another notably unexplored area in the Hippocratic ethic is the social responsibility of the physician. Its emphasis on the welfare of the individual patient is exemplary, and this is firmly explicated in the oath and elsewhere. Indeed, in *Precepts* this respect for the individual patient is placed at the very heart of medicine: "Where there is love of one's fellow man, there is love of the Art." [9]

As Ford has shown, today too the physician's sense of responsibility is directed overwhelmingly toward his or her own patient. [10] This is one of the most admirable features of medicine, and it must always remain the central ethical imperative in medical transactions. But it must now be set in a context entirely alien to that in which ancient medicine was practiced. In earlier eras the remote effects of medical acts were of little concern, and the rights of the individual patient could be the exclusive and absolute base of the physician's actions. Today, the growing interdependence of all humans and the effectiveness of medical techniques have drastically altered the simplistic arrangements of traditional ethics. The aggregate effects of individual medical acts have already changed the ecology of humanity. Every death prevented or life prolonged alters the number, kind, and distribution of human beings. The resultant competition for living space, food, and conveniences already imperils our hope for a life of satisfaction for all.

Even more vexing questions in social ethics are posed when we attempt to allocate our resources among the many new possibilities for good inherent in medical progress and technology. Do we pool our limited resources and manpower to apply curative medicine to all now deprived of it or continue to multiply the complexity of services for the privileged? Do we apply mass prophylaxis against streptococcal diseases, or repair damaged valves with expensive heart surgery? Is it preferable to change cultural patterns in favor of a more reasonable diet for Americans or develop better surgical techniques for unplugging fat-occluded coronary arteries? Every health planner and concerned public official has his or her own set of similar questions. It is clear that we cannot have all these things simultaneously.

This dimension of ethics becomes even more immediate when we inquire into the responsibility of medicine for meeting the urgent sociomedical needs of large segments of our population. Can we absolve ourselves from responsibility for deficiencies in distribution, quality, and accessibility of even ordinary medical care for the poor, the uneducated, and the disenfranchised? Do we direct our health care system to the care of the young in ghettos and underdeveloped countries or to the affluent aged? Which course will make for a better world? These are vexing questions of the utmost social concern. Physicians have an ethical responsibility to raise these questions and, in answering them, to work with the community in ordering its priorities to make optimal use of available medical skills.

It is not enough to hope that the good of the community will grow fortuitously out of the summation of good acts of each physician for his or her own patients. Societies are necessary to insure enrichment of the life of each of their members. But they are more than the aggregate of persons within them. As T. S. Eliot puts it, "What life have you if you have not life together? There is no life that is not in community." [11]

Society supports doctors in the expectation that they will direct themselves to socially relevant health problems, not just those they find interesting or remunerative. The commitment to social egalitarianism demands a greater sensitivity to social ethics than is to be found in traditional codes. Section ten of the American Medical Association Principles of Medical Ethics (1946) explicitly recognizes the profession's responsibility to society. But a more explicit analysis of the relationships of individual and social ethics should be undertaken. Medicine, which touches on the most human problems of both the individual and society, cannot serve human beings without attending to both their personal and communal needs.

This is not to say that medical codes or physicians are to set social priorities. Clearly, individual physicians cannot quantitate the remote effects of each of their medical acts. Nor should they desert their patients to devote themselves entirely to social issues. They cannot withhold specific treatment in hope of preventing some future perturbation of human ecology. Nor can society relegate solely to physicians such policy questions as how and for whom the major health effort will be expended.

In these matters physicians serve best as expert witnesses, providing the basis for informed public decisions. They must lead in pointing out deficiencies and raising the painful matter of choices. At the same time, each doctor must honor his or her traditional contract to help his or her own patient. Doctors cannot allow the larger social issues to undermine that solicitude. Ethically responsive doctors will thus find themselves more and more at the intersection of social and individual ethical values, impelled to act responsibly in both spheres. The Hippocratic ethic and its later modifications were not required to confront such paradoxes. Today's conscientious physicians are very much in need of an expanded ethic to cope with their double responsibility to the individual and to the community.

The institutionalization of all aspects of medical care is an established fact. With increasing frequency, the personal contract inherent in patient care is made with institutions, groups of physicians, or teams of health professionals. Patients now often expect the institution or group to select their physician or consultant and to assume responsibility for the quality and quantity of care provided.

Within the institution itself, the health care team is essential to the practice of comprehensive medicine. Physicians and nonphysicians now cooperate in providing the spectrum of special services made possible by modern technology. The responsibility for even the most intimate care of the patient is shared. Some of the most important clinical decisions are made by team members who may have no personal contact at all with the patient. The team itself is not a stable entity of unchanging composition. Its membership changes in response to the patient's needs, and so may its leadership. Preserving the traditional rights of the patient, formerly vested in a single identifiable physician, is now sometimes spread anonymously over a group. Competence, confidentiality, integrity, and personal concern are far more difficult to assure with a group of diverse professionals enjoying variable degrees of personal contact with the patient.

No current code of ethics fully defines how the traditional rights of the medical transaction are to be protected when responsibility is diffused within a team and an institution. Clearly, no health profession can elaborate such a code of team ethics by itself. We need a new medical ethic which permits the cooperative definition of normative guides to protect the person of the patient served by a group, none of whose members may have sole responsibility for care. Laymen, too, must participate, since boards of trustees set the overall policies which affect patient care. Few trustees truly recognize that they are the ethical and legal surrogates of society for the patients who come to their institutions seeking help.

Thus, the most delicate of the physician's responsibilities, protecting the patient's welfare, must now be fulfilled in a new and complicated context. Instead of the familiar one-to-one unique relationship, physicians find themselves coordinators of a team, sharing with others some

of the most sensitive areas of patient care. Physicians are still bound
to see that group assessment and management are rational, safe, and
personalized. They must especially guard against the dehumanization
so easily and inadvertently perpetrated by a group in the name of
efficiency.

Doctors must acquire new attitudes. Since ancient times, they have
been the sole dominant and authoritarian figures in the care of their
patients. They have been supported in this position by traditional ethics.
In the clinical emergency, their dominant role is still unchallenged, since
they are well trained to make quick decisions in ambiguous situations.
What they are not prepared for are the negotiations, analysis, and ultimate compromise fundamental to group efforts and essential in non-
emergency situations. A whole new set of clinical perspectives must be
introduced, perspectives difficult for the classically trained physician to
accept, but necessary if the patient is to benefit from contemporary
technology and organization of health care.

A central aim of the oath and other ethical treatises is to protect the
patient and the profession from quackery and incompetence. In the
main, competence is assumed as basic in fulfillment of the Hippocratic
ideal of *primum non nocere*. In places, more specific admonitions are to
be found. Thus, in *Law*, "Medicine is the most distinguished of all the
arts, but through the ignorance of those who practice it, and those who
casually judge such practitioners, it is now of all arts by far the least
esteemed." [12] The author of this treatise thus succinctly expressed the
same concerns being voiced at greater length and with more hyperbole
in our own times. In the treatise on fractures, specific advice is given to
prevent curable cases from becoming incurable, to choose the simpler
treatment, to attempt to help, even if the patient seems incurable, and to
avoid "unnecessary torment." [13] Consultation is clearly advised in *Precepts*. [14] In *Decorum*, frequent visits and careful examination are
enjoined. [15]

The Hippocratic works preach the wholly admirable commonsense
ethos of the good artisan: careful work, maturation of skills, simplicity
of approach, and knowledge of limitations. This was sound advice at a
time when new discoveries were so often the product of speculation
untainted by observation or experience. The speculative astringency of
the Hippocratic ethic was a potent and necessary safeguard against the
quackery of fanciful and dangerous "new" cures.

With the scientific era in medicine, the efficacy of new techniques and
information in changing the natural history of disease was dramatically
demonstrated. Today, the patient has a right to access to the vast stores
of new knowledge useful to medicine. Failure of the physician to make
this reservoir available and accessible is a moral failure. The ethos of

the artisan, while still a necessary safeguard, is now far from being a sufficient one.

Maintaining competence today is a prime ethical challenge. Only the highest standard of initial and continuing professional proficiency is acceptable in a technological world. This imperative is now so essential a feature of the patient-physician transaction that the ancient mandate "Do no harm" must be supplemented: "Do all things essential to optimal solution of the patient's problem." Anything less makes the doctor's professional declaration a sham and a scandal.

Competence now has a far wider definition than in ancient times. Not only must physicians encompass expertly the knowledge pertinent to their own field, but they must be the instrument for bringing all other knowledge to bear on their patient's needs. They now function as one element in a vast matrix of consultants, technicians, apparatus, and institutions, all of which may contribute to a patient's well-being. They cannot provide all these things themselves. To attempt to do so is to pursue the romantic and vanishing illusion of the physician as Renaissance man.

The enormous difficulties of its achievement notwithstanding, competence has become the first ethical precept for the modern physician after integrity. It is also the prime humane precept and the one most peculiar to the physician's function in society. Even the current justifiable demands of patients and medical students for greater compassion must not obfuscate the centrality of competence in the physician's existence. The simple intention to help others is commendable but, by itself, not only insufficient but positively dangerous. What is more inhumane or more a violation of trust than incompetence? The consequence of a lack of compassion may be remediable, while a lack of competence may cost the patient a chance for recovery of life, function, and happiness. Clearly, medicine cannot attain the ethical eminence to which it is called without both compassion and competence.

Within this framework, a more rigorous ethic of competence must be elaborated. Continuing education, periodic recertification, and renewal of clinical privileges have become moral mandates, not just hopeful hortatory devices dependent upon individual physician responses. The Hippocratic ethic of the good artisan is now just the point of departure for the wide options technology holds out for individual and social health.

The one-to-one patient-to-physician relationship so earnestly extolled for centuries makes patients almost totally dependent upon their physician for entry into the vast complex of potentially useful services. We cannot leave to fortune or statistics the possibility that patients' choice of a physician might impede their access to all they need for optimal care. We must surround this one-to-one relationship with the safeguards of a corporate responsibility in which the whole profession dedicates itself to protecting the patient's right to competent care.

The whole of the Hippocratic corpus, including the ethical treatises, is the work of many authors writing in different historical periods. Thus, the ethical precepts cannot be considered the formal position of a profession in today's sense. There is no evidence of recognition of true corporate responsibility for larger social issues or of sanctions to deter miscreant members. Indeed, in *Law* there is a clear lament for the lack of penalties to restrain or punish the unethical physician: "medicine is the only art which our states have made subject to no penalty save that of dishonor. And dishonor does not wound those who are compacted of it." [16] Again, in *Precepts,* "Now no harm would be done if bad practitioners received their due wages. But as it is, their innocent patients suffer, for whom the violence of their disorder did not appear sufficient without the addition of their physician's inexperience." [17]

The Greek physician seems to have regarded himself as the member of an informal aristocratic brotherhood in which each individual was expected to act ethically and to do so for love of the profession and respect for the patient. His reward was *doxa,* a good reputation, which in turn assured a successful practice. There is notably no sense of the larger responsibilities as a profession for the behavior of each member. Nowhere stated are the potentialities and responsibilities of a group of high-minded individuals to effect reforms and achieve purposes transcending the interests of individual members. In short, the Greek medical profession relied on the sum total of individual ethical behaviors to assure the ethical behavior of the group.

This is still the dominant view of many physicians in the Western world who limit their ethical perspectives to their relationships with their own patients. Medical societies do censure unethical members with varying alacrity for the grosser forms of misconduct or breaches of professional etiquette. But there is as yet insufficient assumption of a corporate and shared responsibility for the actions of each member of the group. The power of physicians as a polity to effect reforms in quality of care, its organization, and its relevance to the needs of society is as yet unrealized.

Yet many of the dimensions of medical ethics touched upon in this essay can only be secured by the conscious assumption of a corporate responsibility on the part of all physicians for the final pertinence of their individual acts to promote better life for all. There is the need to develop, as it were, a functioning ethical syncytium in which the actions of each physician would touch upon those of all physicians and in which it is clear that the ethical failings of each member would diminish the stature of every other physician to some degree. This syncytial framework is at variance with the traditional notion that all physicians act as individuals and are primarily responsible only to themselves and their patients.

This shift of emphasis is dictated by the metamorphosis of all professions in our complex, highly organized, highly integrated, and egalitarian social order. For most of its history medicine has existed as a select and loosely organized brotherhood. For the past hundred years in our country, it has been more formally organized in the American Medical Association and countless other professional organizations dedicated to a high order of individual ethics. A new stage in the evolution of medicine as a profession is about to begin as a consequence of three clear trends.

First, all professions are increasingly being regarded as services, even as public utilities, dedicated to fulfilling specific social needs not entirely defined by the profession. Professionals themselves will acquire dignity and standing in the future, not so much from the tasks they perform, but from the intimacy of the connection between those tasks and the social life of which the profession is a part. Second, the professions are being democratized, and it will be ever more difficult for any group to hold a privileged position. The automatic primacy of medicine is being challenged by the other health professions whose functions are of increasing importance in patient care. This functionalization of the professions tends to emphasize what is done for a patient and not who does it. Moreover, many tasks formerly performed only by physicians are now being done by other professionals and nonprofessionals. Last, the socialization of all humanity affects the professions as well. Hence, the collectivity will increasingly be expected to take responsibility for how well or poorly the profession carries out the purposes for which it is supported by society.

These changes will threaten medicine only if physicians hold to a simplistic ethic in which the agony of choices among individual and social values is dismissed as spurious or imaginary. Physicians are the most highly educated of health professionals. They should be first to take on the burdens of a continuing self-reformation in terms of a new ethos—one in which the problematics of priorities and values are openly faced as common responsibilities of the entire profession. We must recognize the continuing validity of traditional ethics for the personal dimensions of patient care and their inadequacy for the newer social dimensions of health in contemporary life. It is the failure to appreciate this distinction that stimulates so much criticism of the profession at the same time that individual physicians are highly respected.

What are some of the ethical problems and social responsibilities which are best assured by a corporate posture? We mention but a few as examples, especially those outlined earlier in this essay.

In a technical society with knowledge increasing exponentially, all members of a profession cannot attain the same degree of competence. The whole body of physicians must assume responsibility for guaranteeing to society the highest possible competence in each member. A most effective way to assure this is for each professional group to require, as some already have, the periodic demonstration of continued proficiency as a first condition for continuing membership in the profession. Physicians should take leadership in requiring relicensure and recertification, set the standards of performance, and insist on a remedial and not a punitive approach for those who need refurbishment of their knowledge to qualify for recertification. Implicit in this idea is the possibility that at some point each of us may fail to qualify for reasons such as age, illness, or loss of interest. A profession sensitive to its ethical responsibilities cannot tolerate fading competence, even for reasons beyond the physician's control. Instead, it must provide opportunities for remediation or for alternate, more suitable functions within medicine. Surely the wide range of uses of a medical education will assure a useful place for almost all physicians.

A most potent way to assure competence is to insist that all physicians practice within a context of competent colleagues and peer surveillance. It is an ethical responsibility of the whole profession to see that every licensed physician is a member of a hospital staff. The privilege of using a hospital is primarily a privilege for the patient, not the doctor. To deprive any licensed physicians, because of training, economics, race, or other reasons, of hospital privilege is to deprive their patients and to perpetrate a social injustice. We also thereby lose the best chance to help physicians improve themselves by contact with their colleagues and with institutional standards as well as the informal network of teaching that links physicians together when they can discuss their cases with one another. No rationalization based on economics or professional prerogatives can excuse our profession from its ethical responsibility to enable every practitioner to participate in the mainstream of medical care, in the hospital and the medical school as well. This responsibility should extend to the osteopathic as well as the allopathic physician.

Once every physician is on a hospital staff, there is much the profession can do to develop a context within which competence becomes a value of prime importance. Some institutional mechanisms for review of certain aspects of competence already exist in tissue and utilization committee, though these first steps are not universally applied with sufficient vigor. A well-functioning drug information center in every hospital, a rigorous pharmacy and therapeutics committee, critical reviews of diagnostic accuracy and work-up, comparison of practices against national standards—these are examples of further institutional devices we should insist upon as ethical imperatives. Ultimately, all physicians should have available for their own edification a computerized record of their diagnostic acumen, therapeutic practices, complications, and autopsy correlations. The essential matter is not the specific mechanisms used, but acceptance of the dictum that the competence of each member of the group is, in some real sense, the responsibility of all.

These measures can easily be discounted as repressive, regimentalizing infringements of professional freedom. Or, in a more enlightened ethical view, they can be the practical expression of corporate acceptance of the necessity of workable mechanisms to ensure competence in a technological society. Is there a real ethical choice? The patient, after all, has no means whereby he or she can judge the competence of the services rendered. Individual physicians and the profession owe the patient every possible safeguard. When these are not forthcoming, they will be imposed by a public demanding more accountability in medicine and every other sphere of life.

One of the gravest and most easily visible social inequities today is the maldistribution of medical services among portions of our population. This is another sphere in which the profession as a whole must assume responsibility for what individual physicians cannot do alone. The civil rights movement and the revolt of the black and minority populations have punctuated the problem. Individual physicians have always tried to redress this evil, some in heroic ways. Now, however, the problem is a major ethical responsibility for the whole profession; we cannot dismiss the issue. We must engender a feeling of ethical diminution of the entire profession whenever there are segments of the population without adequate and accessible medical care. This extends to the provision of primary care for all, insistence on a system of coverage for all communities every hour of the day, proper distribution of the various medical specialties and facilities, and a system of fees no longer based on the usual imponderables but on more standardized norms.

Fulfilling such ethical imperatives is sure to cause discomfort for the doctor as well as some loss of privileges and even of remuneration. But unless there is corporate concern translated into corporate action and self-imposed responsibilities, restrictive legislation to achieve these ends seems certain. To an ethically perceptive profession, such legislation should not only be unnecessary, it should be a scandal. It is intrinsic to the very purposes of medicine that physicians exhibit the greatest sensitivity to any social injustice directly related to their mandate in society. The lack of this corporate sensitivity has been acutely perceived by some of today's students and has seriously disaffected them with medical education and practice.[18] We hope, when they assume leadership of the profession, that they will feel these ethical discontinuities as clearly as they do now. If tomorrow's physicians practice what they now preach to their elders, they will indeed expand the ethical responsibilities of our profession into new and essential dimensions. To do so, they will need to supplement traditional medical ethics with a corporate ethical sense as we have just described it.

There are, perforce, reasonable limits to the social ills to which the individual physician and the profession can be expected to attend as physicians. Some have suggested that medicine concern itself with the Vietnam War, the root causes of poverty, environmental pollution, drugs, housing, and racial injustice. It would be difficult to argue that all of these social ills are primary ethical responsibilities of individual physicians or even of the profession. To do so would hopelessly diffuse medical energies and manpower from their proper object—the promotion of health and the cure of illness. The profession can fight poverty, injustice, and war through medicine.

A distinction, therefore, must clearly be made between physicians' primary ethical responsibilities, which derive from the nature of their profession, and those which do not. All physicians must strike for themselves an optimal balance between professional and civic responsibilities. This will depend upon their energy, capabilities, the nature of their specialty, their family responsibilities, and other factors. The extremes of this choice are dangerous: a narrowly technical life, or a free-floating social concern which at best is neurotic and ineffectual and at worst can seriously compromise competence. Ever present is the seductive hubris to which physicians are especially susceptible—the assumption of some special authority or capability in the resolution of all social issues.

It becomes a matter of prime ethical concern for each physician consciously to establish some hierarchy of values and priorities which will define his or her individual and social ethical postures. The ethical responsibilities of the professional group should be broad; those of the individual may of necessity be narrow. Is there some reasonable order of values in the maze of conflicting duties thrust upon physicians today? We will examine this question from the point of view of the clinician.

Surely the first order of responsibility for clinicians must remain with the patients they undertake to treat. Here, the moral imperatives are clear: competence of the highest order, integrity, compassion.

These are continued in traditional medical ethics and can be made more relevant to our times by extension in some of the directions indicated earlier in this essay. To fail in this realm is to violate the trust underlying the personal relationship which characterizes medical care. Nothing is more unconscionable or socially unacceptable.

Only when this first order of ethical requirements has been met can individual physicians address themselves to a second order of responsibilities. These are generally of two kinds: those which arise from medical progress—like human experimentation and genetic and behavioral modification—and those which bear directly on the condition of life of the community—population control, eradicating malnutrition, assurance of accessibility, comprehensive health care for all citizens, abortion, drugs, and so on. Of the two sets, the latter are more directly related to the daily work of the practitioner and pose ethical issues of an immediate nature, since they flow so directly from his or her first-order responsibilities.

In these matters, physicians can indeed act as leaders, sensors of unmet needs, and expert witnesses in constructing feasible solutions. They can mobilize their county and state society to assume corporate responsibility for distributing physicians, for mandating coverage of all communities, perhaps experimenting with use of nonphysicians. Physicians can use their authority as clinicians to underline needs for improvement of services and facilities in their community. If they clearly focus on patient and community health and not on their own prerogatives, there can be no more effective voice in initiating reforms.

The third order of responsibilities—those more properly related to the physician—are among the most crucial for modern individuals. Yet they are usually outside the physician's prerogatives and distant from his or her direct function in society. Important as they are, these issues—poverty, war, racism—require knowledge doctors must acquire. If these are doctors' major concerns, they should make no pretense at also being clinicians, or they will become clinicians in the most limited sense. Medical education and experience make a legitimate base for service in new fields or social and political action, but they do not legitimatize the neglect of clinical competence in individual medical acts. This distinction needs careful scrutiny by those who would have physicians cure the accumulated social ills of our times and who upbraid them for their failures to do this and to maintain professional competence as well. "If you try to act beyond your powers, you not only disgrace yourself in it, but you neglect the part which you could have filled with success." [19]

Individual physicians can, and indeed should, limit their ethical pretensions. The profession as a body can but should not. Physicians as a group must assume ethical responsibility which may bind each physician. The profession, as we have shown, must attempt to do as a body what individuals cannot do by themselves—namely, span the full range of ethical imperatives. The profession is bound to assume responsibility for the ethical behavior of its members, for setting the context which best guarantees good behavior and taking sanctions against members who fall from their high estate while at the same time effecting their rehabilitation. Physicians as individuals may eschew certain responsibilities as inappropriate, but the profession cannot.

Herein, then, lies the final guarantee for the patient and the community: the interplay of ethical responsibilities for each individual physician and of the whole body of physicians. Each physician must consciously define on several levels his or her personal moral responsibilities. The profession simultaneously must call for deep involvement of its members at all levels of ethical responsibility—the individual clinical medical transaction, the social consequences of medical acts and medical progress, the quality and availability of medical services, and the duties of its educated group to engage in the larger social issues confronting contemporary humanity. This reinforcement of the ethical perspective of the individual physician by a heightened ethical perception of the community of physicians is an essential ingredient of any professional ethical framework which hopes to cope with the current flux in values and goals afflicting modern society.

What will happen to the conscience and the values of the individual physician if the claims of society and the profession are given new ethical force? The law can insist that confidences be revealed in the interest of justice; if abortion is legalized, the physician as agent of society will be expected to provide this service; the same is true if euthanasia, personality and behavioral modification, and chemical sterilization should become public mandates. How shall we balance social and public mandates against the conscience of the individual physician? How will we safeguard the integrity of the physician's own values?

We have a terrifying example of the inability of physicians to withstand social pressures in the acts of unmitigated evil perpetrated by the physicians in German prison camps. These physicians abdicated conscience and choice so thoroughly that they participated in the most reprehensible acts, convinced that they were innocent bystanders. The individual conscience simply ceased to exist, and the individual physician became a mindless cipher. They were willingly conscripted into that "auxiliary bureaucracy" which Gabriel Marcel so scathingly deplores in *Man against Mass Society.*[20]

The very horror of this possibility should underscore how essential is the defense of the mind, conscience, and values of the individual physician and his or her patient in any system of medicine, ethics, or political organization. This is all the more reason for an axiologic approach, which always calls for an orderly analysis of the values underlying moral choices. The highest ethical call is still that of the conscience of an individual human person, a conscience which must be prepared at all times to take issue with social directives, corporate agreements, and political pressures. The dignity and the worth of the human being he or she treats must still remain the beacon that guides the physician's conscience in the ethical night before us. Marcel pinpoints this duty so peculiar to our times: "It is within the scope of each of us, within his own proper field, in his profession, to pursue an unrelaxing struggle for man, for the dignity of man against everything that today threatens to annihilate man and his dignity." [21]

We have attempted a brief analysis of some of the limitations and omissions in traditional medical ethics as embodied in the Hippocratic corpus and its later exemplifications. These limitations are largely in the realm of social and corporate ethics, realms of increasing significance in an egalitarian, highly structured, and exquisitely interlocked social order.

The individual physician needs more explicit guidelines than traditional codes afford to meet today's new problems. The Hippocratic ethic is one of the most admirable codes in the history of man. But even its ethical sensibilities and high moral tone are insufficient for the complexities of today's problems.

An evolving, constantly refurbished system of medical ethics is requisite in the twentieth century. An axiologic, rather than a deontologic, bias is more in harmony with the questions raised in a world society whose values are in continual flux and reexamination. There is ample opportunity for a critical reappraisal of the Hippocratic ethic and for the elaboration of a fuller and more comprehensive medical ethic suited to our profession as it nears the twenty-first century. This fuller ethic will build upon the noble precepts set forth so long ago in the Hippocratic corpus. It will explicate, complement, and develop those precepts, but it must not be delimited in its evolution by an unwarranted reluctance to question even so ancient and honorable a code as that of the Hippocratic writings.

## Notes

1. American Academy of Arts and Sciences, *Proceedings* 98, no. 2 (1969); E. D. Pellegrino, "The Necessity, Promise, and Dangers of Human Experimentation," in *Experiments with Man,* World Council Studies, no. 6 (New York: World Council of Churches, Geneva, and Friendship Press, 1969); "New Dimensions in Legal and Ethical Concepts for Human Research," *Annual of the New York Academy of Arts and Sciences* 169 (1970): 293–593.

2. Ibid.; E. F. Torrey, *Ethical Issues in Medicine* (Boston: Little, Brown and Co., 1968); E. D. Pellegrino, *Medical Progress and Human Values: The Changing Dimensions of Medical Ethics* (Cambridge, Mass.: Harvard University Press, in press).

3. H. E. Sigerist, *The History of Medicine,* vol. 11 (New York: Oxford University Press, 1961), 260, 298; W. A. Heidel, *Hippocratic Medicine: Its Spirit and Method* (New York: Columbia University Press, 1941), 149.

4. W. H. S. Jones, ed. and trans., *Hippocrates* (Cambridge, Mass.: Harvard University Press, 1923), vol. 1, 229–301.

5. Ibid., vol. 2, 263–265.

6. Ibid., vol. 1, 299–301.

7. C. Leake, ed., *Percival's Medical Ethics* (Baltimore: William Wilkins, 1927), 291.

8. Jones, *Hippocrates,* vol. 2, 263–265.

9. Ibid., vol. 1, 299–301.

10. Ford et al., *The Doctor's Perspective* (New York: Year Book, 1967).

11. T. S. Eliot, "The Rock," in *The Complete Poems and Plays, 1909–1950* (New York: Harcourt and Brace, 1952), 101.

12. Jones, *Hippocrates,* vol. 2, 263–265.

13. M. Michler, "Medical Ethics in Hippocratic Bone Surgery," *Bulletin of the History of Medicine* 42 (1968): 297–311.

14. Jones, *Hippocrates,* vol. 1, 299–301.

15. Ibid., vol. 2, 263–265.

16. Ibid.

17. Ibid., vol. 1, 299–301.

18. C. Truett, A. W. Douville, B. Fagel, et al., "The Medical Curriculum and Human Values," *Journal of the American Medical Association* 209 (1969): 1341–1345.

19. W. Oates, ed., *The Stoic and Epicurean Philosophers* (New York: Modern Library, 1957), 480.

20. G. Marcel, *Man against Mass Society* (Chicago: Henry Regnery, 1962), 180.

21. Ibid.

# 5. *The Golden Rule and the Cycle of Life*

Erik H. Erikson

As the George W. Gay Lecturer of 1962, I took advantage of my position to offer a few insights from my study of life histories, a field of study first inspired by a series of physicians (from Sigmund Freud to William James and Henry Murray) who became psychologists and who created, out of the study of cases, the study of lives. The insights advanced will, it is hoped, prove to be relevant to "wise and proper conduct," even though the only kind of ethical investment to be recommended is that of one generation to the next.

My base line is the Golden Rule, which advocates that one should do (or not do) to another as one would be (or not be) done by. Systematic students of ethics often indicate a certain disdain for this all-too-primitive ancestor of loftier and more logical principles. Yet this rule has marked a mysterious meeting ground between ancient peoples separated by oceans and eras and is a theme hidden in the most memorable sayings of many thinkers.

I would like to take the Talmudic version of the Golden Rule for my opening: "What is hateful to yourself, do not to your fellow man." The Talmud adds, "That is the whole of the Torah and the rest is but commentary. Go and learn it." The rule in this form, as critics have never tired of pointing out, is only the rock bottom of moral prudence. But then it was so stated by Rabbi Hillel in answer to an unbeliever's challenge that he be told the whole of the Torah while he stood on one foot. Pressed for brevity, the great rabbi put basic things first. If he added that the rest was but commentary, nobody acquainted with the Jewish way of life would mistake but commentary for merely commentary, for surely sometimes the ongoing commentary is the very life of a rule.

The Golden Rule obviously concerns itself with one of the very basic paradoxes of human existence. All individuals call their own a separate body, a self-conscious individuality, and a personal awareness of the cosmos; and yet they share this world as a reality also perceived and judged by others and as an actuality within which they must commit themselves to ceaseless interaction. To identify self-interest and the interest of other selves, the rule alternately employs the method of warning, "Do as you would be done by." For psychological appeal, some versions rely on the minimum of egotistic prudence, already quoted, while others demand a maximum of altruistic sympathy. It must be admitted that the formula "Do not to others what if done to you would cause you pain" does not presuppose much more than the mental level of the small child who desists from pinching when it gets pinched in return; while mature insight and more is assumed in the saying "No one is a believer until he loves for his brother what he loves for himself." Of all the versions, however, none commits us as unconditionally as "Love thy neighbor as thyself." It even suggests a true love of ourselves.

I will not (I could not) involve us in comparative religion by tracing the versions of the rule to various world religions; no doubt in translation all of them have become somewhat assimilated to our biblical versions. Yet the basic formula seems to be universal, and it reappears in an astonishing number of the most revered sayings of our civilization, from St. Francis' prayer to Kant's moral imperative to Lincoln's single political creed: "As I would not be slave, I would not be master."

The variations of the rule have, of course, provided material for many discussions on ethics weighing the soundness of the logic implied and measuring the degree of ethical nobility reached in each. My field of inquiry, the study of life histories, suggests that I desist from arguing relative logical merit or spiritual worth, and instead relate some variations in moral and ethical sensitivity to successive stages in the development of human conscience; in the framework of the life cycle, the most primitive rules and the most exalted may well prove to be necessary to each other.

I almost decided to discuss medical ethics and not medical morality. The implication is clear: those who know what is legal and what is moral or immoral have not necessarily learned thereby what is ethical. Highly moralistic people can do unethical things, while an ethical person's involvement in immoral doings becomes by inner necessity an occasion for tragedy. The dictionary, our first refuge from ambiguity, in this case only compounds it: morals and ethics are defined as synonyms and antonyms of each other. In other words, they are the same with a difference—a difference which I intend to emphasize.

I would propose that we consider moral rules of conduct to be based *sake of duty* on a fear of threats to be forestalled—outer threats of abandonment, punishment, public exposure, or a threatening inner sense of guilt, shame, or isolation. In contrast, I would consider ethical rules to be based on a love of ideals to be striven for, ideals which hold up to us some highest good, some definition of perfection, and some promise of self-realization. This differentiation is, I think, substantiated by developmental observations, and the developmental principle is the first of those which will represent for us the kind of insight which we have gained from the study of life histories.

All that exists layer upon layer in an adult's mind has developed step by step in the growing child's, and the major steps in the comprehension of what is considered good behavior in one's cultural universe are related—for better and for worse—to different stages in individual maturation. The response to a moral tone of voice develops early. The small child, so limited to the intensity of the moment, somehow must learn the boundaries marked by don'ts. Here, cultures have a certain leeway in underscoring the goodness of one who does not transgress or the evilness of one who does. But the conclusion is unavoidable that children can be made to feel evil and that adults continue to project evil on one another and on their children far beyond the call of rational judgment.

Before discussing this early moral sense in more detail, let me mention the later steps which I will differentiate from it: they are the development of an ideological sense in adolescence and an ethical sense in young adulthood. The imagery of steps, of course, is useful only where it is to be suggested that one item precedes another in such a way that the earlier one is necessary to the later ones and that each later one is of a higher order. But development is more complex, especially since all manner of step formations take place simultaneously and in not-too-obvious synchronization.

To return to the moral sense, psychoanalytic observation first established in a systematic fashion what certain eastern thinkers have always known; namely, that radical division into good and bad can be a sickness of the mind. It has traced the moral scruples and excesses of the adult to the childhood stages in which guilt and shame are ready to be aroused and are easily exploited. It has named and studied the superego, which hovers over the ego as the inner perpetuation of the child's subordination to the restraining will of his elders. The voice of the superego is not always cruel and derisive, but it is ever ready to become so whenever the precarious balance which we call a good conscience is upset, at which times the secret weapons of this inner governor are revealed: the brand of shame and the bite of conscience. Are these "caused" or merely accentuated by the pressure of parental and communal methods, by the threat of loss of affection, corporal punishment, public shaming? Or are they by now a proclivity for self-alienation which has become a part— and to some extent a necessary part—of our evolutionary heritage?

All we know for sure is that our moral proclivity does not develop without the establishment of some chronic self-doubt and some truly terrible—even if mostly submerged—rage against anybody and anything that reinforces such doubt. The "lowest" in us is thus apt to reappear in the guise of the "highest": irrational and prerational combinations of goodness, doubt, and rage can reemerge in the adult in those malignant forms of righteousness and prejudice which we may call moralism. In the name of high moral principles we can employ all the vindictiveness of derision, torture, and mass extinction. One surely must come to the conclusion that the Golden Rule was meant to protect us not only against our enemies' open attacks, but also against our friends' righteous encroachments.

Lest this view, in spite of the evidence of history, seem too "clinical," we turn to the science of evolution, which in the last few decades has joined psychoanalysis in recognizing the superego as an evolutionary fact—and danger. The developmental principle is thus joined by an evolutionary one. Waddington even goes so far as to say that superego rigidity may be an overspecialization in the human race, like the excessive body armor of the late dinosaurs. In a less grandiose comparison he likens the superego to "the finicky adaptation of certain parasites which fits them to live only on one host or animal." In recommending his book *The Ethical Animal* (in addition to the works of J. Huxley and G. G. Simpson), I must admit that his terminology contradicts mine. He calls the awakening of morality in childhood a proclivity for "ethicizing," whereas I would prefer to call it moralizing. As do many animal psychologists, he dwells on analogies between the very young child and the young animal instead of comparing, as I think we must, the young animal with the preadult human, including the adolescent.

I cannot dwell here on the new insights regarding the cognitive and emotional gains of adolescence which enable the young, often only after a severe bout with moralistic regression, to envisage more universal principles of a highest human good. The adolescent learns to grasp the flux of time, to anticipate the future in a coherent way, to perceive ideas, and to assent to ideals—to take, in short, an ideological position for which the younger child is cognitively not prepared. In adolescence, then, an ethical view is approximated, but it remains susceptible to an alternation of impulsive judgment and odd rationalization. It is, then, as true for adolescence as it is for childhood that our way stations to maturity can become fixed, can become premature platforms for future regression, in the individual person and in masses of individuals.

The moral sense, in its perfections and its perversions, has been an intrinsic part of our evolution, while the sense of ideological rejuvenation has pervaded our revolutions, both with prophetic idealism and with destructive fanaticism. Adolescent humans, in all their sensitivity to the ideal, are easily taken in by the promise of a new and arrogantly exclusive identity.

The true ethical sense of the young adult at its best encompasses moral restraint and ideal vision while insisting on concrete commitments to those intimate relationships and work associations by which we can hope to share a lifetime of productivity and competence. But young adulthood engenders its own dangers. It adds to the moralist's righteousness—and to the ideologist's repudiation of all otherness—the territorial defensiveness of one who has appropriated and staked out an earthly claim and who seeks eternal security in the superidentity of organizations. Thus, what the Golden Rule at its highest has attempted to make all-inclusive, tribes and nations, castes and classes, moralities and ideologies have consistently made exclusive again—proudly, superstitiously, and viciously denying the status of reciprocal ethics to those "outside."

If I have so far underscored the malignant potentials of our slow maturation, I have done so not in order to dwell on a kind of dogmatic pessimism which can emerge all too easily from clinical preoccupation and often leads only to anxious avoidances. I know that our moral, ideological, and ethical propensities can find, and have found on occasion, a sublime integration in individuals and in groups who were both tolerant and firm, flexible and strong, wise and obedient. Above all, we have always shown a dim knowledge of our better potentialities by paying homage to those purest leaders who taught the simplest and most inclusive rules for an undivided humanity. But we have also persistently betrayed them, on what passed for moral or ideological grounds, even as we are now preparing a potential betrayal of all human heritage on scientific and technological grounds in the name of that which is considered good merely because it can be made to work—no matter where it leads.

We begin to see where it may lead. But only in our time, and in our very generation, have we come to view with a historical start the obvious fact that in all of previous history the rule, in whatever form, has comfortably coexisted with warfare. A warrior, all armored and spiked and set to do to another what he fully expected the other to be ready to do to him, saw no ethical contradiction between the rule and his military ideology; he could, in fact, grant to his adversary a respect which he hoped to earn in return. This tenuous coexistence of ethics and warfare may outlive itself in our time. The military mind may well come to fear for its historical identity when technical mass annihilation replaces tactical warfare. The Golden Rule of the nuclear age, which is, "Do not unto others unless you are sure you can do them in as totally as they can do you in," creates not only an international deadlock but a profoundly ethical one as well.

One wonders, however, whether this deadlock can be broken by even the most courageous protest, the most incisive interpretation, or the most prophetic warning—a warning of catastrophe of such immensity that most of us will ignore it as we ignore certain death and have learned to ignore the monotonous prediction of hell. It seems instead that only an ethical orientation, a direction for vigorous cooperation, can free today's energies from their bondage in armed defensiveness. We live at a time in which, for all the species-wide destruction possible, we can think for the first time of a species-wide identity, of truly universal ethics, such as have been prepared in the world religions, in humanism, and by some philosophers. Ethics cannot be fabricated; they can only emerge from an informed and inspired search for a more inclusive human identity which a new technology and a new world image make possible as well as mandatory.

Our sociogenetic evolution is about to reach a crisis in the full sense of the word: a crossroads offering one path to fatality and one to recovery and further growth. Artful perverters of joy and keen exploiters of strength, we have learned to survive "in a fashion," to multiply without food for the multitudes, to grow up healthy without reaching personal maturity, to live well but without purpose, to invent ingeniously without aim, and to kill grandiosely without need. But the processes of sociogenetic evolution also seem to promise a new humanism: our acceptance—as an evolved product as well as a producer and a self-conscious tool of further evolution—of the obligation to be guided in our planned actions and chosen self-restraints by our knowledge and insights. In this endeavor, then, it may be of a certain importance to learn to understand and to master the differences between infantile morality, adolescent ideology, and adult ethics. Each is necessary to the next, but each effective only if they eventually combine in that wisdom which, as Waddington puts it, "fulfills sufficiently the function of mediating evolutionary advance."

At the point when one is about to end an argument with a global injunction of what we must do, it is good to remember Blake's admonition that the common good readily becomes the topic of "the scoundrel, the hypocrite, and the flatterer," and that those who would do some good must do so in "minute particulars." And indeed, I have so far spoken only of development and the evolutionary principle, according to which the propensity for ethics grows in the individual as part of an adaptation roughly laid down by evolution. Yet, to grow in the individual, ethics must be generated and regenerated in and by the sequence of generations. This generational principle we must now make more explicit.

Let me make an altogether new start here; let us look at scientific humans in their dealings with animals. Harry Harlow's studies on the development of affection in monkeys are well known. He did some exquisite experimental and photographic work attempting, in the life of laboratory monkeys, to "control the mother variable." He took monkeys from mothers within a few hours after birth, isolated them, and left them with "mothers" made out of wire, metal, wood, and terry cloth. A rubber nipple somewhere in their middles emitted piped-in milk, and the whole contraption was wired for body warmth. All the "variables" of this mother situation were controlled: the amount of rocking, the degree of "body warmth," and the exact incline in the maternal body necessary to make a scared monkey feel safe and comfortable. Years ago, when this method was presented as a study of the development of affection in monkeys, the clinician could not help wondering whether this was monkey affection or a fetishist addiction to inanimate objects. And, indeed, while these laboratory-reared monkeys became healthier and healthier and much more trainable in technical know-how than the inferior monkeys brought up by mere monkey mothers, they became at the end what Harlow calls "psychotics." They sat passively, they stared vacantly, and some did something terrifying: when poked they bit themselves and tore at their own flesh until the blood flowed. They had not learned to experience "the other," whether as mother, mate, child—or enemy. Only a tiny minority of the females produced offspring, and only one of them made an attempt to nurse hers. But science remains a wonderful thing. Now that we have succeeded in producing "psychotic" monkeys experimentally, we can convince ourselves that we have at last given scientific support to severely disturbed mother-child relationships as causative factors in human psychosis.

It speaks for Harry Harlow's methods that what they demonstrate is unforgettable. At the same time, they lead us to that borderline where we recognize that the scientific approach toward living beings must be with concepts and methods adequate to the study of ongoing life, not of selective extinction. I have put it this way: one can study the nature of things by doing something to them, but one can only learn about the essential nature of beings by doing something with them or for them. This, of course, is the principle of clinical science. It does not deny that one can learn by dissecting the dead, or that an animal or a human can be motivated to lend circumscribed parts of his or her being to an experimental procedure. But for the study of those central transactions which are the carriers of sociogenetic evolution and for which we must take responsibility in the future, the chosen unit of observation must be the generation, not the individual. Whether an individual animal or human being partook of the stuff of life can only be tested by the kind of observation which discerns his or her ability to transmit life—in some essential form—to the next generation.

One remembers here the work of Konrad Lorenz and the kind of "interliving" research which he and others have developed, making, in principle, the life cycle of certain selected animals part of the same environment in which observers live their own life cycle, and studying their role as well as the animals, taking their chances with what their ingenuity can discern in a setting of sophisticated naturalist inquiry. One remembers also Elsa the lioness, a foundling who was brought up in the Adamson household in Kenya. There, the mother variable was not controlled, it was in control. Mrs. Adamson and her husband even felt responsible for putting grown-up Elsa back among the lions and succeeded in sending her back to the bush, where she mated and had cubs and yet came back from time to time (accompanied by her cubs) to visit her human foster parents. In our context we cannot fail to wonder about the built-in "moral" sense that made Elsa respond—and to respond in very critical situations, indeed—to the words, "No, Elsa, no," if the words came from human beings she trusted. Yet even with this built-in "moral" response and with a lasting trust in her foster parents (which she transmitted to her wild cubs), she was able to live as wild lions do. Her mate, however, never appeared; he apparently was not too curious about her folks.

The point of this and similar stories is that our habitual relationship to what we call beasts in nature and "instinctive" or "instinctual" beastliness in ourselves may be highly distorted by thousands of years of superstition; there may be resources for peace even in our "animal nature" if we will only learn to nurture nature as well as master her. Today, we can teach a monkey, in the very words of the Bible, to "eat the flesh of his own arm," even as we can permit "erring leaders" to make of all humanity the "fuel of the fire." Yet it seems equally plausible that we can let our children grow up to lead "the calf and the young lion and the fatling together"—in nature and in their own nature.

To recognize one of our prime resources, however, we must trace back our individual development to our premoral days—our infancy— which are marked by basic trust, an overall attitude integrating what in the newborn organism reaches out to the caretakers and establishes with them what we will now discuss as mutuality. The failure of basic trust and of mutuality has been recognized in psychiatry as the most far-reaching development failure, undercutting all development.

I would call mutuality a relationship in which partners depend on each other for the development of their respective strengths. A baby's first responses can be seen as part of an actuality consisting of many details of mutual arousal and response. While the baby initially smiles at a mere configuration resembling the human face, adults cannot help smiling back, filled with expectations of a "recognition" which they need to secure from the new being as surely as it needs them. The fact is that the mutuality of adult and baby is the original source of the basic ingredient of all effective as well as ethical human action: hope. As far back as 1895, Freud, in his first outline of a "Psychology for Neurologists," counterpoints to the "helpless" newborn a "help-rich" (*hilfreich*) adult and postulates that their mutual understanding is "the primal source of all moral motives." Should we, then, equip the Golden Rule with a principle of mutuality, replacing the reciprocity of both prudence and sympathy?

Parents dealing with a child will be strengthened in their vitality, in a sense of identity, and in a readiness for ethical action by the very ministrations by means of which they secure to the child his or her vitality, a future sense of identity, and an eventual readiness for ethical action. On this mutuality, then, all ethical potentialities are built—and we know how tragic and deeply pathogenic its absence can be in children and parents who cannot arouse and cannot respond.

But we should avoid making a new utopia out of the mother-child relationship. The paradise of early childhood must be abandoned—a fact which we have not yet learned to accept. The earliest mutuality is only a beginning and leads to more complicated encounters as both the child and his or her interaction with a widening cast of persons grow more complicated. I need only point out that the second basic set of vital strengths in childhood (following trust and hope) is autonomy and will, and it must be clear that a situation in which the child's willfulness faces the adult's will is a different proposition from that of the mutuality of instilling hope. Yet any adults who have managed to train a child's will must admit—for better or for worse—that they have learned much about themselves and about will that they never knew before, something which cannot be learned in any other way. Thus all growing individuals' developing strength dovetails with the strengths of an increasing number of persons arranged about them in the social orders of family, school, community, and society. These orders, in turn, safeguard themselves by formalizing the Golden Rule in a hierarchy of institutions. But all orders and rules are kept alive by those "virtues" of which Shakespeare (in what appears to me to be his passionate version of the rule) says that "shining upon others [they] heat them and they retort that heat again to the first giver."

With such high encouragement I will try to formulate my amendment to the Golden Rule. I have been reluctant to come to this point; it has taken thousands of years and much linguistic acrobatics to translate the rule from one era to another and from one language into another, and at best one can only confound it again in a somewhat different way.

It would, at any rate, seem irrelevant to formulate any new or better do's or don't's than the rule already implies in its classical forms. Rather, I would advocate a general orientation not too narrowly hemmed in by scruples and avoidances and not too exclusively guided by high promises and rewards. This orientation has its center in whatever activity or activities give us the feeling, as William James put it, of being "most deeply and intensely active and alive." In this, James promises, each will find his or her "real me"; but, I would now add, he or she will also acquire a conviction that truly ethical acts enhance a mutuality between the doer and the other, a mutuality which strengthens the doer even as it strengthens the other. Thus, the "doer unto" and "the other" are one deed. Developmentally, this means that doers are activated in whatever strength is appropriate to their age, stage, and condition, even as they activate in others the strength appropriate to their age, stage, and condition.

Our next step is to demonstrate that the inequality of parent and child or, better, the uniqueness of their respective positions which has served as our model so far has significant analogies in other situations in which uniqueness depends on a divided function. Here, eventually, we may come closer to an application of our amendment of the rule to medical ethics as well.

But there is one more principle which must be added to the developmental one, to mutuality, and to the generational principle. I already implied it in the term "activate," and I would call it the principle of active choice. It is, I think, most venerably expressed in St. Francis' prayer: "Grant that I may not so much seek to be consoled as to console; to be understood as to understand; to be loved as to love, for it is in giving that we receive." Such commitment to a decisive initiative in love is, of course, contained in the admonition to "love thy neighbor." It is not in our domain, however, to discuss that religious frontier of existence where we expect to derive our most decisive ethical initiative from a highest grace. Yet I think that we can recognize in these exalted words a psychological verity which determines that only those who approach an encounter in an active and giving attitude (consciously and unconsciously), rather than in a demanding and dependent one, will be able to make of that encounter what it can become.

To return to particulars, I will attempt to apply my amendment to the diversity of function in the two sexes. I have not dwelt so far on this most usual subject of a psychoanalytic discourse, sexuality. So much of this otherwise absorbing part of life has in recent years become stereotyped, and not the least among the terminological culprits to be blamed for this sorry fact is the psychoanalytic term "love object." For the word "object" in Freud's theory has been taken too literally by many of his friends and by most of his enemies. (Moralistic critics do delight in misrepresenting a man's transitory findings as his ultimate "values.") The fact is that Freud, on purely conceptual grounds and on the basis of his scientific training, pointed out that drives have objects; but he never said, and he certainly never advocated, that men or women should treat one another as objects on which to live out their sexual desires.

Instead, his central theory of a mutuality of orgasm which combines strivings of sexuality and of love points, in fact, to one of those basic mutualities in which a partner's potency and potentialities are activated even as he or she activates the other's potency and potentialities. Freud's theory implies that a man will be more a man to the extent to which he makes a woman more a woman—and vice versa—because only two uniquely different beings can enhance their respective uniqueness for one another. A "genital" person in Freud's sense is thus more apt to act in accordance with Kant's version of the Golden Rule; namely, that one should so act as to treat humanity (whether in his or her person or in another) "always as an end, and never only as a means." What Freud added, however, was a methodology which opens to our inquiry and to our influence the powerhouse of inner forces which provide the shining heat for our strength—and the wavering smoke of our weaknesses.

I cannot leave the subject of the two sexes without a word on the uniqueness of women. One may well question whether the oldest versions of the rule meant to acknowledge women as partners in the golden deal; and today's study of lives still leaves quite obscure the place of women in what is most relevant to men. True, women are being granted equality of political rights and the recognition of a certain sameness in mental and moral equipment. But what they have not begun to earn, partially because they have not cared to ask for it, is the equal right to be effectively unique and to use hard-won rights in the service of what they uniquely represent in human evolution.

One senses today the emergence of a new feminism as part of a more inclusive humanism. This coincides with a growing conviction—highly ambivalent, to be sure—that the future of humanity cannot depend on men alone and may well depend on the fate of a mother variable uncontrolled by technological man. The resistance to such a consideration always comes from men and women who are mortally afraid that by emphasizing what is unique one may tend to reemphasize what is unequal. The study of life histories certainly confirms a far-reaching sameness in men and women insofar as they express the mathematical architecture of the universe, the organization of logical thought, and the structure of language. But such study also suggests that while boys and girls can think and act and talk alike, they naturally do not experience their bodies (and thus the world) alike: one could illustrate this by pointing to sex differences in the structuralization of space in the play of children. But I assume here that a uniqueness of either sex will be granted without proof, and that the "difference" acclaimed by the much-quoted Frenchman is not considered a mere matter of anatomical appointments for mutual sexual enjoyment, but a psychological difference central to two great modes of life, the paternal and the maternal modes.

The study of creative men reveals that only a vital struggle makes it possible for them to reconcile in themselves the paternal and the maternal dimensions of all mental productivity. It may well be that there is something in woman's specific creativity which has only waited for a clarification of her relationship to masculinity (including her own) in order to assume her share of leadership in those fateful human affairs which so far have been left entirely in the hands of gifted and driven men, and often of men whose creativity eventually has yielded to ruthless self-aggrandizement. Humanity now obviously depends on new kinds of social inventions and on institutions which guard and cultivate that which nurses and nourishes, cares and tolerates, includes and preserves. Mere conquest and invention alone, and more expansion and organization, will make life more exciting but not more livable. And if my amendment to the rule suggests that one sex enhances the uniqueness of the other, it also implies that each, to be really unique, depends on a mutuality with an equally unique partner: only when women dare to assume the motherhood of man may men be emboldened to overcome the boyhood of history.

By now one may well have reached the conclusion that my discursiveness was intended to leave me little time for the problem of medical ethics. However, medical ethics can only be a variation of a universal theme, and it was necessary to establish the general context within which

I could hope to give a slightly different emphasis to a subject so rich in tradition.

There is a very real and specific inequality in the relationship of doctor and patient in their roles of knower and known, helper and sufferer, practitioner of life and victim of disease and death, for which reason medical people have their own and unique professional oath and strive to live up to a universal ideal of "the doctor." Yet the practice of the healing arts permits extreme types of practitioners: from the absolute authoritarian over homes and clinics to the harassed servant of demanding humanity; from the sadist of mere proficiency to the effusive lover of all (well, almost all) his or her patients.

Here, too, Freud has thrown intimate and original light on the workings of a unique relationship. His letters to his friend and mentor Fliess illustrate the singular experience which made him recognize in his patients what he called "transference"; that is, patients' wish to exploit sickness and treatment for infantile and regressive ends. Moreover, Freud recognized a "countertransference" in the healer's motivation to exploit the patients' transference and to dominate or serve, possess or love them to the disadvantage of their true function. He made systematic insight into transference and countertransference part of the training of the psychoanalytic practitioner. I would think that all of the motivations necessarily entering so vast and intricate a field could be reconciled in a Golden Rule amended to include a mutuality of divided function. Each specialty and each technique in its own way permits the doctor to develop as a practitioner and as a person, even as the patient is cured as a patient and a person. A real cure transcends the transitory state of patienthood; it is an experience which enables the cured patient to develop and to transmit to home and neighbor an attitude toward health which is one of the most essential ingredients of an ethical outlook. This variation on the overall theme of an amended rule is all I can offer in the framework of this discussion; intensive discussion will, I hope, lead to more detailed and more concrete matter vital to medical practice.

Beyond this, can the healing arts and sciences contribute to a new ethical outlook? This question always recurs in psychoanalysis and is usually disposed of with Freud's answer that the psychoanalyst represents the ethics of scientific truth only and is committed to studying ethics (or morality) in a scientific way. Beyond this, he leaves *Weltanschauungen* (ethical world views) to others.

It seems to me, however, that the clinical arts and sciences, while employing the scientific method, are not defined by it or limited by it. Healers are committed to a highest good, preserving life and furthering well-being. They need not prove scientifically that these are, in fact, the highest good; rather, they are precommitted to their basic proposition while investigating what can be verified by scientific means. This, I think, is the meaning of the Hippocratic Oath, which subordinates all medical method to a humanist ethic. True, individuals can separate their personal, professional, and scientific ethics, seeking fulfillment of needs in personal life, the welfare of others in their profession, and, in their research, truths independent of personal preference or service. However, there are psychological limits to the multiplicity of values anyone can live by, and, in the end, not only practitioners but also their patients and research depend on a certain unification of temperament, intellect, and ethics; this unification clearly characterizes great doctors.

While it is true, then, that as scientists we must study ethics objectively, we are, as professional individuals, committed to unifying personality, training, and conviction which alone will help us to do our work adequately. At the same time, as transient members of the human race, we must record the truest meaning of which the fallible methods of our era and the accidental circumstances of our existence have made us aware. In this sense, there is (and always has been) not only an ethic governing clinical work and a clinical approach to the study of ethics, but also a contribution to the ethics of the healing orientation. Healers, in addition, have now committed themselves to prevention on a large scale, and they cannot evade the question of how to assure ethical vitality to all lives saved from morbidity and early mortality.

And now a final word on what is, and will be for a long time to come, the sinister horizon of the world in which we all study and work: the international situation. Here, too, we cannot afford to live for long with a division of personal, professional, and political ethics—a division endangering the very life which our professions have vowed to keep intact and thus cutting through the very fiber of our personal existence. But again, I can offer you only another variation of the theme and propose, in all brevity, that what has been said here about the relationships of parent and child, of man and woman, and of doctor and patient may have some application to the relationships of nations to each other, nations which by definition are units at different stages of political, technological, and economic transformation. I know that it is all too easy for us to believe that nations thus engaged should treat one another (or at least that we should treat others) with a superior educative or clinical attitude. This is not what I mean. The point is, again, not one of underscored inequality but one of respected uniqueness within historical differences. Insofar as a nation thinks of itself as a collective individual it may well learn to visualize its task as that of maintaining international relations of mutuality. For the only alternative to armed competition seems to be the effort to activate in the historical partners what will strengthen them in their historical development even as it strengthens the actors in their own development—toward a common future identity. Only thus can we find a common denominator in the rapid change of technology and history and transcend the dangerous imagery of victory and defeat, of subjugation and exploitation, which is the heritage of a fragmented past.

Does this sound utopian? I think, on the contrary, that all of what I have said is already known in many ways, is being expressed in many languages, and is practiced on many levels. At our historical moment it becomes clear in a most practical way that the doer of the Golden Rule, and he or she who is done by, is the same individual, is humanity.

Those of clinical background, however, must not lose sight of a dimension which I have taken for granted in what I have said. While the Golden Rule in its classical versions prods us to strive consciously for a highest good and to avoid mutual harm with a sharpened awareness, our insights assume an unconscious substratum of ethical strength and, at the same time, unconscious arsenals of destructive irrationality. The last century has traumatically expanded our awareness of the existence of motivations stemming from our animal ancestry, economic history, and inner dividedness; but it has also created methods of productive self-scrutiny. It will be the task of the next generation to begin to integrate such new awareness with the minute particulars not only of advancing proficiency but also of ongoing mutuality by which alone our ready rage is neutralized.

It does not seem easy to speak of ethical subjects without indulging in some moralizing and ideologizing. As an antidote I will repeat the final words of the quotation from the Talmud with which I began. It does not say: "Here is the rule; go, and act accordingly." It says: "Go, and learn it." Here lies our challenge.

# 6. Narcissus, Pogo, and Lewis Thomas' Wager

Roger J. Bulger

> I have seen the enemy
> and he is us.
>
> —Pogo

Any analysis of ethical issues in health policy has to begin with the distressing admission that our civilization's fundamental values are now in question and that what social critics and psychiatrists are calling "narcissism" is undermining our society. As I tried to get excited about attempting an explication of one or another of the ethical issues in health policy, I found myself returning to four major words—"society," "health," and "human values"—and a growing feeling that there are higher-priority questions our nation and civilization must settle before the ethical issues in health policy can be sensibly addressed. Thus, I am led to offer a personal view of our situation, painting with broad strokes from a variety of sources in the hope that there might be some implications for action.

## Narcissism

Just as in the 1960s, when many of society's critics and pundits talked of cultural sadness or cultural boredom as a leading symptom or even as a disease afflicting our civilization, the decade of the 1970s seems to have belonged to Narcissus. Christopher Lasch, Aaron Stern, and Robert Coles have been among those who have written about narcissism and American society. Such considerations seem inevitably to lead to comparisons between the current situation in the modern Western world and the fall of the Roman Empire.

Will and Ariel Durant, in their multivolume work *The Story of Civilization,* make the following comments:

> A great civilization is not conquered from without until it has destroyed itself within. The essential causes of Rome's decline lay in her people, her morals, her class struggle, her failing trade, her bureaucratic despotism, her stifling taxes, her consuming wars. . . . The cause, however, was no inherent exhaustion of the soil, no change in the climate, but the negligence and sterility of harassed and discouraged men. . . . The dole weakened the poor, luxury weakened the rich. . . . Moral decay contributed to the dissolution. . . . The virile character that had been formed by arduous simplicities and a supporting faith relaxed in the sunshine of wealth and the freedom of unbelief; men had now, in the middle and upper classes, the means to yield to temptation, and only expediency to restrain them. Urban congestion multiplied contacts and frustrated surveillance; immigration brought together a hundred cultures, whose differences rubbed themselves out into indifference. Moral and esthetic standards were lowered by the magnetism of the mass; and sex ran riot in freedom while political liberty decayed. . . . The potential causes of decay were rooted in one fact—that increasing despotism destroyed the citizen's civic sense and dried up statesmanship at its source. Powerless to express his political will except by violence, the Roman lost interest in government and became absorbed in his business, his amusements, his legion, or his individual salvation.[1]

Aaron Stern, a Connecticut psychoanalyst, published in 1979 a book titled *Me—The Narcissistic American,* which addresses many of these issues.

> No society has ever survived success. The record of history is clear. . . . The Roman Empire provides a richly detailed descrip-

tion of the decline of a great society. The symptoms of its fall centered around a critical schism between the older and younger generations. It was reflected among the young by an increase in drug usage, by a growing experimentation in homosexuality and bisexuality, and, perhaps most symptomatic of all, by a strident demand for more leisure that was accompanied by an unwillingness to accept responsibility for government, family, and other institutions.[2]

Christopher Lasch has written perhaps the deepest and most provocative interpretation of this issue in his book *The Culture of Narcissism: American Life in an Age of Diminishing Expectations.* Among many trenchant and incisive observations Professor Lasch makes of our culture, he reverses Stern's approach of beginning with the individual and working up to society and proposes that society expresses its culture through the individual:

> Every society reproduces its culture—its norms, its underlying assumptions, its modes of organizing experience—in the individual, in the form of personality. As Durkheim said, personality is the individual socialized. The process of socialization, carried out by the family and secondarily by the school and other agencies of character formation, modifies human nature to conform to the prevailing social norms.[3]

In this view, if narcissism is widespread amongst our citizenry, it must be inherent in our societal agencies of character formation.

It does not take much stretching of the mind to appreciate from these three passages why many thoughtful critics of American society are worried that we are following the same trajectory as did the late Roman Empire. One wonders where we can find a societal booster rocket to alter our collective course.

In a recent article titled "Civility and Psychology," Robert Coles made some additional observations about the destructive side of the widespread epidemic of the "me-first" syndrome:

> Psychology, in this instance, means a concentration, persistent, if not feverish, upon one's thoughts, feelings, wishes, worries— bordering on, if not embracing solipsism: The self as the only or main form of (existential) reality. . . . Backward souls from New Mexico and Mississippi talked about "kin" or "land" as of transcendental importance (even as God and later the nation-state once were held in such commanding esteem). Today it is "groups" that

matter, people who know how to talk and talk. . . . The hallmark
of our time seems to be lots of psychological chatter, lots of self-
consciousness, lots of "interpretation." As the saying goes, "Let
it all hang out," and then we'll talk about it. . . . A crude kind
of popularized psychology has become the moral standard many,
many people rely upon. . . . The self is our guide, our standard—
those psychological "needs" we experience, those psychological
"passages" through which we journey, those "emotions" we boast-
fully proclaim to each other.[4]

Thus, it seems sadly true that many of our young people are seeking
their maturity and identity in a society in which cultural boredom has
been replaced by a consuming interest in oneself. The famous line attributed to Louis XIV, "L'état c'est moi!" (I am the state) could fairly be
argued to have become the paradoxical watchword of increasing millions
of Americans.

Aleksandr Solzhenitsyn, in an article in *Foreign Affairs*, presented his
compellingly stark view of Soviet imperialism, made all the more depressing by recent world events. Solzhenitsyn seems to hold little hope
for us as a society, as he says:

The West simply does not want to believe that the time for sacrifices has arrived; it is simply unprepared for sacrifices. Men who
go on trading right until the first salvo is fired are incapable of sac-
rificing so much as their commercial profits: They have not the wit
to realize that their children will never enjoy these gains, that today's illusory profits will return as tomorrow's devastation. The
Western allies are maneuvering to see who can sacrifice the least.
Behind all this lies that sleek god of affluence which is now proclaimed as the goal of life, replacing the high-minded view of the
world which the West has lost.[5]

## Role of Health Professionals

It might now be appropriate to consider how health professionals and
scientists, through their various enterprises and activities, contribute,
often unconsciously, to these trends. First of all, the health and medical
establishment quite appropriately is aggressively pushing the benefits to
personal health of scientific research, medical interventions, and preventive measures; most recently, we are increasingly active in convincing
the public to adopt improved behaviors and life-styles better adapted to
promoting "health," both physical and mental. Unfortunately, implicitly
and occasionally explicitly, these efforts reinforce the narcissism in all

of us. All too often I catch myself saying to people: "Good health is your greatest blessing," when if I really thought about it I might say: "Good health is one of your three or four greatest blessings." As health professionals and biobehavioral scientists, we know that the more we get the public concerned and involved with their health, the more supportive they will be of our enterprises—and that can be an insidious force if we do not act to put personal health in proper perspective.

Lewis Thomas makes this point:

> Americans are obsessed with their health, and—paradoxically—it's because we have become a great deal healthier in the last half century. . . . Today, having realized that it is possible to influence health and to prevent or cure disease, we now view disease itself as less acceptable. . . . Some of the media emphasis has been useful, but it has its negative side: It tends to leave the impression that we are constructed as a kind of imperfect organism—fallible and fragile and likely to collapse unless we are propped up by what it is now fashionable to call the health care system. . . . There's an awful lot of talk these days implying that it is abnormal to be unhappy. You read things that suggest that if you're unhappy you ought to go see a doctor and if you're depressed, as everybody is from time to time, you are ill. There's a whole new profession of people who advise other people on how to live a life—as though you could take courses in some part of the university and learn how to live wisely and sagaciously and end up being happy or avoid being unhappy. This has been greatly overdone. . . . There's a lot of genuine mental illness. I don't have any questions that schizophrenia and manic-depressive psychoses are real things. But it worries me that people, especially the young are being brought up to believe that if they're unhappy, they ought to go see a counselor and get what's called guidance.[6]

In those comments, Thomas introduced the second way in which the health professions contribute to cultural narcissism; that is, by establishing and maintaining an inappropriate role for the professions in our society.

Lasch points out that the same forces in our culture that have turned the worker into a consumer have worked to convert the citizen into a client.[7] The professions, by his reckoning, have helped create the destructive transference of responsibility from the individual and the family to the "helping professions" and to society. In Lasch's view of our society, it has become axiomatic that individuals are ineffective in helping themselves with serious problems, whereas the professions claim the ability to make significant contributions at almost any level. For Professor Lasch, our narcissistic society is a dying society that celebrates personal citizen incompetence.

A third way in which the health professions tend to support society's narcissistic gestalt is our penchant for approaching our problems and most important issues by plebiscite. The interest in self has become such a dominant force in our social research, as we go from poll to poll to determine what "we" think, feel, or divine, that it sometimes seems to me that we are guided by only two principles: the first is that a poll shall ultimately determine the truth, and the second is that all "taboos" are wrong and shall be avoided, a principle that may be rooted in the idea that any rule that interferes with self-expression or self-fulfillment is wrong. Once the American public believes it is afflicted with a taboo, it seeks to extirpate it as expeditiously as possible.

## Taboos and Trends

Take, for example, the precept that physicians or other legitimate healers should not have sexual relations with their patients. Not long ago, two investigators carried out some surveys in Orange County, California questioning both practicing physicians and medical students about their attitudes and behavior regarding this precept. The findings indicated that a small but significant minority of practicing physicians admitted to having had sexual relations with their patients and did not see anything wrong with it; a larger minority of fourth-year medical students and a still larger minority of first-year medical students did not, in prospect, see anything wrong with such behavior when they themselves became physicians. The authors then concluded that there was clearly a trend of which those charged with developing the medical ethical codes should take note, recognize, and, by implication, use as a basis for changing the existing interdiction against such behavior.

Another currently developing scenario has to do with incest. A study has now been done to show that incest is a more common phenomenon than was previously thought. Furthermore, a significant proportion of parents and children who have never practiced incest have admitted to being tempted by the thought. Just recently, another study claimed that in families where incest is practiced, there is a surprisingly small proportion that showed any serious psychological damage to the participants. One may anticipate that the next study will claim that 99.4 percent of incestuous relationships are fun and seem to predispose to better sexual performance in later life; it will then be clear that the home is, as with religious instruction, the best place to learn practical sex. If not actually promoted, incest will next become a morally neutral phenomenon, and another taboo will have been destroyed.

In both of these instances, an ethical or moral precept or code gets examined in the medical literature from the point of view of impact on individual health or feelings. If there is no definable damage to the individual discovered in these researches, then the power of science will have seemed to stand opposed to certain moral and ethical codes; we all tend to yield to "expert" opinion and the findings of "science." The interdictions against sex with patients or with family members have many roots other than the simple concern for the person's health or feelings. If society ever decides to drop these rules or principles, one hopes such an action would follow ethical, anthropological, social, and legal analyses and debates. My fear is that these codes will simply slide away with the "knowledge" that "lots of people are trying whatever it is, and it doesn't seem to hurt them." One cannot help but wonder where we think we are going.

Robert Coles, in reviewing Gay Talese's book *Thy Neighbor's Wife*, made the following comments relevant to my argument:

> Gay Talese, the well-known journalist . . . now offers us a report on just how far some of us have willingly, gladly strayed not only from 19th-century morality, but from the kind most of the 20th century has taken for granted. . . . We are given, really, a number of well-told stories, their social message cumulative: A drastically transformed American sexuality has emerged during this past couple of decades. . . . At one point, however, and none too soon, the author reminds us . . . that there are "millions of Americans" who have been quite religious, "whose marriages were unadulterous," and who want no part of the activity that has been strongly enhanced by "all the various social, legal and biological devices which allow increased sexual freedom." [8]

But, it turns out, this freedom seems to do little to improve on the human condition; the folks who fully express themselves sexually seem no less venal and trite than the rest of us. And Coles asks a much more important question:

> What happened to the children whose parents got caught up in the "growth centers" and "people changes" and "love nests" this book describes? We hear little about those boys and girls; they seem set aside, forgotten, handed over (we are several times told) to a succession of babysitters—as if love for a "neighbor's wife" matters

> more by far than the welfare of mere children. . . . What happens
> to a culture, a civilization, when sexual fantasies become for in-
> creasing numbers a reigning preoccupation? . . . As philosophers
> once knew to put it—and would that they did so more often these
> days: what is the meaning of life, and how ought one to live it?[9]

One must note, however, that any honest appraisal of our current fall-
ing out with the traditional Judeo-Christian ethic must consider the disillusionment during the past quarter-century of increasing numbers of
people with an overly simplistic view of the universe, governed by a
caring God interested in keeping the righteous safe and ultimately in
maintaining the natural world as humankind's preserve. The cumulative
impact of the horrors and disappointments of Auschwitz, Hiroshima,
Korea, Vietnam, Watergate, and so many others of the past forty years
has led us to a serious questioning of an ethic and world view at once
too simple, too repressive, and, in the end, no longer sufficiently convincing to demand our allegiance. Meanwhile, as "Big Science" ex-
ploded, the conventional wisdom seemed to be that we were closing
in on all the mysteries of nature and the universe. And there seemed
nothing in all of this to suggest that humanity was anything more than
a passing chance in what had turned out to be a rather minor biological
parade between two ice ages. As our majority belief in that old cosmology crumbled, there was nothing to replace it to give meaning to individual or national life, and it may thus have been anticipated that
narcissism would be a likely result.

This is not meant to imply that the general attack on meaningless
rules, regulations, habits, and taboos is all bad. Clearly, many positive things have come from the sexual revolution. We can expect major
changes in our society as the role of women continues its evolution. It
is certain that the open airing of the subject of death and the care of the
dying has produced some significant improvements over the past twenty
years, not only in the attitudes of health professionals but also among
the public at large. There is obviously great advantage to destroying the
negative charges attached to words like epilepsy, cancer, alcoholism,
leprosy, tuberculosis, and so forth, so that victims of these diseases
are not laden with additional problems from the society in which they
must live.

Nevertheless, it seems too easy to destroy old myths, symbols, and
values; more often we must ask, what is there to replace them? The Harris Poll? Such a poll may uncover what the majority of a sample of the
population may believe—and that all too often becomes labeled as "the
majority belief," which may be further refined and studied and reformu-
lated by one leader or another until it becomes a new policy. That new

policy usually removes more constraints or restrictions from acceptable norms of human behavior and seldom seems to project a new or heightened sense of values.

As a last example of how the health establishment may be contributing to the "narcissistic society," we must consider the contract or the terms that define the relationship between the physician and patient. Most critics, friendly enough to support the validity and concept of an oath, seem to agree that currently acceptable oaths are overly paternalistic and have other shortcomings that must be addressed if we hope to establish a more appropriate and creative modern-day contract between patient and physician. Without going into the detail this subject deserves, let me assert that a restructured contract could do much to influence the behavior and expectations of both patients and professionals, more effectively restoring to the former an opportunity to become competent citizens— guardians of their own destinies.

Ludwig Eichna's recently published reflections on medical education are not unrelated to how the physician-patient relationship will work in the future and indicate that in his experience the "me-first" approach has become a subconscious part of the fabric of the socialization and education of medical students and resident physicians:

> Two forces are responsible for the teaching of bad medical ethics: schools, directly and society, indirectly but powerfully. . . . As for the schools, the bad teaching begins in college, where unethical competition among premedical students indoctrinates the me-first state of mind. This attitude persists in medical school in the students' actions toward patients. Patients are looked on not as ill people but almost as impersonal beings that exist for the students' own development. Faculty confirm this attitude in their teaching. They too have an ingrained blind spot. . . . All will contest this charge, but let each stand aside and look carefully at his or her own actions; each will be surprised by the validity of the charge. . . . We are not industrialists. We do not conduct a business. We sell no product to consumers. We are doctors. We take care of, and we care for, patients. We must be mindful of cost, yes, but the patient comes first.[10]

Other critics might add that in those instances when the patient or the student is not "first" in medical education, the faculty seems to be. It is clear that this trend or tendency could be systematically eliminated if medical educators agreed to discourage the me-first approach and to promote patient-centeredness as the primary behavioral objective of every step in the educational process. I suspect that similar behavioral changes might be equally appropriate and desirable among the faculties and curricula of other health professional schools.

Looking to the future, we may ask, What hope is there? What may we expect? Are the doomsayers to be right at last, or can we find hopeful signs anywhere? On the hopeful side, some social scientists say that the age of moral ambiguity in the United States is on the decline. Yankelovich and Lefkowitz, in the prestigious journal *Public Opinion,* recently analyzed existing data regarding the expectations of the American public for the next decade. They concluded that there is a growing acceptance of resource limitation, of the need and even desirability of sacrifice. Furthermore, there is increasing doubt that technology can solve our problems. Finally, they say, "Americans speak enthusiastically about the moral benefits of a simple, nonmaterialistic life. But they have yet to fully incorporate these benefits into either their day-to-day behavior or their practical planning for the future." [11]

Thus, there seems to be an opportunity for thoughtful health establishment leaders to step into a policy leadership role. They can do this first by asserting their values and beliefs and seeking some greater consensus on fundamental societal values.

## Lew Thomas' Wager

Is narcissism our worst disease? I believe it is time we said so, admitted the overmedicalization of society, and proposed that health is not the greatest good.

Can it be that time will end with our generation or our civilization and that a nuclear holocaust will be the end of the line for humanity? Can it be that creation is not still unfolding, that our evolution is not somehow of continuing meaning and purpose to be expressed for thousands of years ahead through the species *Homo sapiens?*

Thomas has come up with a modern version of Pascal's wager. (Blaise Pascal, seventeenth-century French philosopher, when asked to state his position on the existence of God and the eternal life of the soul, indicated that if he expressed his belief in such eternal life and was right, he had everything to gain; whereas if he expressed disbelief and was wrong, he had everything to lose. Therefore, he would wager on God and eternal life.) In a recent speech he stated:

> Today, an intellectually fashionable view of man's place in nature
> is that there is really no great problem: the plain answer is that it
> makes no sense, no sense at all. The universe is meaningless for
> human beings: we bumbled our way into the place by a series of
> random and senseless biological accidents. The sky is not blue: this

is an optical illusion—the sky is black. You can walk on the moon
if you feel like it, but there is nothing to do there except look at the
earth, and when you've seen one earth, you've seen them all. The
animals and plants of the planet are at hostile odds with one another, each bent on elbowing any nearby neighbor off the earth.
Genes, tapes of polymer, are the ultimate adversaries and, by random, the only real survivors. . . . This grasp of things is sometimes presented as though based on science, with the implication
that we already know most of the important knowable matters and
this is the way it all turns out. It is the wisdom of the 20th century,
contemplating as its only epiphany the news that the world is an absurd apparatus and we are stuck with it, and in it. . . . In this cir-
cumstance, we would surely have no obligation except to our
individual selves. . . . I believe something considerably less than
this. I take it as an article of faith that we humans are a profoundly
immature species, only now beginning the process of learning how
to learn. . . . I cannot make my peace with the randomness doctrine: I cannot abide the notion of purposelessness and blind chance
in nature. And yet I do not know what to put in its place for the
quieting of my mind. . . . What I would like to know most about
the developing earth is: Does it already have a mind? Or will it
someday gain a mind, and are we part of that? Are we a tissue
for the earth's awareness? . . . I like this thought, even though I
cannot take it anywhere, and I must say it embarrasses me. I have
that nagging hunch that it is a presumption, a piece of ultimate
hubris. . . . I would like to think that we are on our way to becoming an embryonic central nervous system for the whole system. I
even like the notion that our cities, still primitive, archaic, fragile
structures, could turn into the precursors of ganglia, to be ultimately linked in a network around the planet. But I do worry, from
time to time, about that other possibility: that we are a transient
tissue, replaceable, biologically representing a try at something
needing better means of perfection. . . . But, at better times, remembering how skilled our species is with language and metaphor . . . and remembering that nature is by nature parsimonious,
tending to hang on to useful things when they really do work, I
have hopes for our survival into maturity, millennia ahead.[12]

   As the world grinds on to a human saturation and growing poverty
and hunger, and if we continue to participate in an affluent subset of human society, must we really accept the ultimate pessimism and cynicism
of widespread narcissism and a modern societal collapse to rival that of
Rome?

If, on the other hand, we are to share Thomas' optimism and are hopeful about humankind and seek to propagate the race, then we must take an active part in dealing with the values we wish to perpetuate. If freedom as we know it in the West is a crucial element, perhaps we should encourage the surgeon general to declare not only that "Narcissism may be our worst national affliction," but also that "Totalitarianism or dictatorship or other serious loss of personal freedoms may be harmful to our health!"

We should perhaps ask more about the value of rules and limits in healthy human behavior, rather than pursuing conscious efforts at their destruction. It may be important to explore in a more systematic way than our behavioral scientists have done in the past the value to the individual's mental health of seeking a goal transcending oneself. How can we obtain a better cultural identity in these fast-changing times, especially an identity that can bind us together in meaningful activity as a society? Must we have a war in order to do the hard things as a nation?

We should encourage policies that favor the young and ensure that all of our children have optimal educational opportunities for growth and development. We should seek to do all in our power to preserve and undergird the integrity of the family unit in our society.

We should take a strong position against nuclear war—just because the bomb has been dropped twice, it does not mean that for the future such interventions should not be treated as chemical and biological warfares now are. Why should we accept so readily the concept of the inevitability of a nuclear holocaust?

We should more clearly enunciate the importance of hope to our way of life. Thus, economic analyses may often indicate that an intervention or set of interventions in the health care system are too costly for the benefits they may produce. Our phenomenal network of tertiary care centers, though highly expensive, offer hope to all who never have to use them, because everyone has the assurance that the technology is there to repair the injured or impaired person should the need arise. In the United States, we pride ourselves on giving people another chance, that we are never out just because we are down, and that the disabled and sick should be given an opportunity to come back. How much is a life worth? is one side of the coin; the other is, How much will we pay for all of us to have hope in the potential for cure or rehabilitation should we become seriously ill? That particular American value—in my view seldom appropriately appreciated and consistently underestimated, especially by health economists and analysts—will be sorely tested in the years ahead, because our capacity to provide expensive technical aids to chronically disabled people will be limited only by the resources we are willing to dedicate to these purposes.

Finally, if we concur with Pogo that we "have seen the enemy and he is us,"—Narcissus—and if we accept the optimism inherent in what I have referred to as Thomas' wager, then the quest for new knowledge must be continually emphasized and supported. The investment in the future that comes from the support of basic research is thus the quintessential expression of an unselfish society willing to sacrifice for the benefit of generations yet unborn.

By way of summary, let me simply state that I find societal narcissism to be the last step before mass cynicism and pessimism deny us a sense of the future. I hope and trust we shall go no further with our narcissism and will actively work to find an individual and collective meaning capable of reconnecting our citizenry with each other and our society. Some of our time-honored and traditional values will help, but surely we shall have to develop new insights and new ways of viewing things. Whatever the relative merits of the various options before us, I will place my money with Lew Thomas', because, among other advantages, his view promises to be so much more fun than the alternatives.

## Notes

1. Will and Ariel Durant, *The Story of Civilization,* vol. 3 (New York: Simon and Schuster, 1944), 665–668.

2. Aaron Stern, *Me—The Narcissistic American* (New York: Ballantine Books, 1979).

3. Christopher Lasch, *The Culture of Narcissism: American Life in an Age of Diminishing Expectations* (New York: W. W. Norton, 1978).

4. Robert Coles, "Civility and Psychology," *Daedalus* 109 (1980): 133–142.

5. Aleksandr Solzhenitsyn, "Misconceptions about Russia Are a Threat to America," *Foreign Affairs* 58 (1980): 797–834.

6. Lewis Thomas, *Atlanta Constitution,* May 3, 1980, 1–3.

7. Lasch, *The Culture of Narcissism.*

8. Robert Coles, *New York Times Book Review,* May 4, 1980, 3.

9. Ibid.

10. Ludwig W. Eichna, "Medical-School Education 1975–1979: A Student's Perspective," *New England Journal of Medicine* 303 (1980): 727–734.

11. D. Yankelovich and B. Lefkowitz, "National Growth: The Question of the '80s," *Public Opinion* (December 1979–January 1980): 44–57.

12. Lewis Thomas, "On the Uncertainty of Science," *Harvard Magazine* (September–October 1980): 19–22.

# 7. *On the Drinking of the Hemlock: Socrates, Semmelweis, and Barbara McClintock*

**Roger J. Bulger**

As I get older and continue to acquire more and more experience, I have come increasingly to be impressed with the importance of character, integrity, and honesty in the evaluation and selection of people at every level. I have also learned that the most trying and difficult challenges in my professional life center on my ability to live up to my own ideals and to preserve, in full, my integrity. Therefore, I found it an easy task to decide that an administrator in the field of higher education should be willing to participate actively in considerations of the subject of honesty and truth in the doing of science.

It is well known that, in the history of large organizations and institutions, both the values held by individuals and the environment in which those individuals operate can change. Such changes may be subtle but may act continuously in the same direction so that over time significant alterations may occur such as to affect the other element (i.e., the environment may change enough to impact the value system of individuals or vice versa); in the case of large organizations or whole segments of

societal expression, like science or the arts, such changes may significantly alter for better or worse the productivity, effectiveness, or impact
of the institution. We are used to the idea nowadays that change is so
rapid in our society that dramatic alterations seem to occur before we
are aware that they have begun. What we used to know but sometimes
seem to forget is that a true history cannot be written intelligently until
enough time has passed to provide a necessary perspective. Thus, for
example, discussions about whether or not there is more or less dishonesty in science now than in the past, whether or not people value integrity less than they used to, and whether therefore the very foundations
of modern science are or are not under more serious threat now than in
earlier times are less relevant than are efforts to understand the basic values of modern science, to combat dishonesty, and to protect and promote the essentials of the proper environment for the flourishing of
science. It is in this spirit that this analysis is undertaken of the interactions among the modern scientist and his or her individual commitment
to the search for new knowledge, the overall scientific and academic environment, and the values of society at large.

I thought it would be useful to begin my brief remarks on honesty and
dishonesty in science by recounting three illustrative events of historic
importance. The first occurred in 1956 in the famous Lido nightclub in
Paris where I was asked to appear with the star magician-comedian. It
happened that as three of us young Americans waited for the show to
begin, we were invited backstage to consider participating in one of the
main acts. We were asked to raise our hands when the audience was so-
licited for volunteers and naturally we were to be the three "plants"
from among the twelve chosen. The comedian explained that he needed
only three collaborators out of twelve volunteers to create the environment sufficient to fool the other nine and the entire audience. As a
sleight-of-hand artist and pickpocket he had no peer and as each volun-
teer came up to the stage he lifted his watch or wallet or keys. The three
plants were prepared for even more startling tricks: I, for example, had
fairly long trousers on, so the fact that I had removed one sock and
given it to the magician before the show was obscured from the audience
until he pulled up my trouser leg and then, with a flourish, removed my
sock from his pocket, convincing most people that he had somehow gotten the sock off my foot in full view of everyone. One of my friends had
his tie cleverly rearranged backstage so that the magician could pull it
off with one quick, clean swipe of his lightninglike hands. The other
had his shirt removed before the show and then carefully laid on his
chest so that it looked perfectly normal, but at the proper time the magician was able to reach under my friend's jacket at his wrist and slowly

pull on the shirt sleeve until the entire shirt emerged in the hand of this worker of wonders—a truly astonishing feat.

But all of this was only a prelude to the final illusion. With great fanfare he announced that he was going to send out a magical electric shock to all twelve of his volunteers through the normal wooden chairs on which we had been sitting at our tables and on which the entire audience sat. The chairs were passed up to the stage and all of us and the audience could see they were simple wooden chairs unconnected to any wires and placed upon a large, bare, wooden stage. The magician had us all sit down on the chairs and explained that whenever he did this show the electricity in his body just built up and surged out to shock the volunteers, never lethally, but at a time he simply couldn't predict. Further, he said that so far this great electrical discharge had never spread off stage to the audience, which nevertheless grew a little more tense. He had prearranged with us that when he said a certain word during his monologue the three of us would leap from our chairs, holding our backsides as though we had suddenly received a mighty electric shock. He told us he had been doing this nightly for several years and that if the plants did their jobs right on cue and together it had never failed that all the other nine would leap up almost instantaneously and many would claim afterward that they indeed had felt a mighty "shock" when, of course, there had been none! At the appointed word, my colleagues and I leaped into the air . . . and the other nine did too, looking like a well-rehearsed set of cheerleaders, to the utter astonishment of the audience. I was next to an American sailor, to whom I shouted over the din, "My God! Did you feel that?" He answered excitedly, "Yeah . . . it felt like I was being electrocuted!" Afterward, in talking with our other friends in the audience, all well educated and highly critical, it became apparent they believed most of what they had seen. It was clear that a clever person could deceive a large audience of smart people, especially when he did things they expected, but even when he did things that are impossible, like pulling a person's shirt off by tugging at the sleeve. This is the flip side of seeking truth; in show business or in science it is relatively easy to perpetrate fraud and deceit.

The second episode is more truly historic and relates to Ignaz Semmelweis, the great Hungarian physician who discovered how to prevent puerperal fever, which in 1848 was responsible for the deaths of 10 to 30 percent of all women who delivered babies in the best European hospitals. Semmelweis decided it was the doctor who was transmitting the disease from patient to patient with his unwashed hands. In 1848 he published the data showing the reduction to virtually zero of the incidence of puerperal fever among his patients through the simple expedient of washing his hands between examinations as he proceeded on his rounds in the hospital wards. His data were clear and uncontestable; year after year he continued to have no or very few maternal deaths, while in the same hospital in Vienna in which he practiced and in hospitals in every major European city the women died by the thousands, until in 1860 other evidence emerged which allowed people to understand why Semmelweis was right and had been right all along. So, after fifteen years of totally unnecessary slaughter, medical practice was brought into line with the observable facts. Shortly thereafter the great Semmelweis died, a broken and discredited person, having been committed by friends to a mental institution, a victim, some people say, of his adherence to the truth despite the absolute blindness of his colleagues to the facts and their subsequent virtual expulsion of Semmelweis from their company of respected professionals and scientists. (Of parenthetic interest is the fact that in 1837 Oliver Wendell Holmes published an article in America exhorting doctors to wash their hands between deliveries. He was totally ignored. His response was to wait ten years and then republish the exact same article in another journal; again he was ignored.) There are many similar though less dramatic examples of scientists uncovering a new kernel of truth only to meet with resistance, denial, or nonrecognition by their peers, whose minds seem closed rather than open. This is not fraud or deceit; rather it is a retardation of progress because of a failure of the basic principle of open-mindedness to new "truths," to which principle in theory all scientists adhere.

Speaking of hidden kernels of truth, probably the most striking recent example of this is the Barbara McClintock story of transposition of genetic material.[1] McClintock, a botanist whose life's work involves classical genetic studies on corn and who was an eventual winner of the Nobel Prize, proposed her theory on transposition in well-documented studies published in the early 1950s. Her work and theory were essentially ignored until Jacob and Monod presented their analogous work on regulator genes in 1960; McClintock did not get full recognition until the dominant, opinion-shaping force of the molecular biologists came to accept the so-called jumping gene concept. As with Semmelweis, a second scientific probe had to occur to make the prior discovery intelligible and therefore acceptable to the scientific establishment.

The third little vignette I'd like to spotlight for your consideration is a commentary on modern American life and standards which I find especially worrisome and threatening. There are a series of advertisements we have all heard on Preparation H, the much heralded treatment for hemorrhoids. The ad begins with a person representing an average American, typical of any one of us, saying to a friend that he or she can't do something because the boss had made some unanticipated demands at work. The announcer chimes in and says, "Mr. Jones is lying! The real reason he can't go is his hemorrhoids are bothering him." The message I get when I hear this ad is not that Preparation H is so effective, but that most people with hemorrhoids (and I presume that means potentially the entire population) are liars and that lying, however innocuous, is now an expected and accepted form of behavior in our society. In effect, we have become a nation of liars. (If that's true, why should I believe what they say about Preparation H?)

"Truth" is the motto of America's first university. As I meandered intellectually through my education (largely taken at that great university), I wondered when I'd recognize and find the truth. When formal education passed and I realized I hadn't found it yet, it occurred to me that the searching might be the key to the problem of life—that the commitment to the search may be the highest calling, or certainly a high calling. As I have grown older I have, from time to time, begun to wonder at the diminishing capacities of my mind and to question my ability to grow in wisdom; while recently, a recurrent image keeps inserting itself into these daydreams of mine, and that is the image of this great brain we each have (by some estimates, the equivalent of a computer the size of the State of Texas and twelve stories high) beginning a gradual but inexorable implosion as it ages with neurons and cells collapsing on one another, becoming enmeshed in new ways and in a more concentrated fashion until, lo and behold, just at the moment of death, as the aging brain finally collapses on itself to the ultimate concentration, the truth emerges and becomes known, especially to the person who has spent a lifetime seeking it.

In a peculiar way this strange image recapitulates a little of what I want to share with you, and that relates to what I perceive to be the emergence of certain intellectual unities and perhaps even of a moral imperative out of the maelstrom of ideas and values that swirl around all of us in modern westernized society. Sometimes it seems to me that modern-day astronomers sound like theologians, physicists talk like philosophers, biologists write like poets and mystics, and, I should like to hope, quite possibly, truth seeking and truth speaking are emerging as unifying values of our society and culture.

Four hundred years before Christ, Socrates, a man with no program, no written record, and no gainful employment, spent his life in dialogue with others, conversing with all who would engage in his persistent questioning and seeking for the truth. He did not pretend to know the truth; in fact, he believed his function was to puncture the illusions of those who thought they did. For his trouble he was condemned to die by a jury of fellow Athenians and, rather than run away, thereby making a mockery of his own steadfast support of the rules and laws of his city,

he drank the poison hemlock, executed by his peers and seemingly ending his life in abject failure because he would not lie. Unaware of the
truth, knowing only that he must keep seeking it and never yield to un-
truthfulness along the way, Socrates sanctified truth seeking and truth
telling by his life and death and in many ways became a kind of secular
patron saint of truth.[2]

Some leading observers worry that the structure of our society is dis-
integrating. George Orwell warned us that 1984 might see a society
grounded upon a system of organized lying. Certainly our ideals and
values are being challenged at every turn. Even in these times of disillusionment, nuclear despair, and information overload, a young plu-
ralistic but democratic society such as ours must consider that there is
one basic undergirding of almost any important relationship between
and among people and institutions, and that underpinning is trust, based
in turn upon honesty and integrity.[3] There are many thoughtful people
who believe that the intent to seek and speak the truth is essential to the
survival of the free world; increasingly, it seems to me this commitment
to truth may be the moral imperative which, potentially, can be adhered
to by every responsible citizen in our diverse society, regardless of his or
her basic philosophic or religious beliefs.

I can only offer a smorgasbord of ideas in support of the centrality of
truth seeking and truth telling to our society's well-being.

Lewis Thomas has made a second career of late in preaching our ignorance in matters scientific to a lay audience. What we know is mi-
nuscule compared to what we can know, and the most important thing
is to recognize our ignorance.[4] Upon this basically Socratic message
Thomas builds his arguments for a greater investment in science.

Sissela Bok, a modern American philosopher and ethicist, recently
has written two books of considerable interest, the first on lying[5] and the
second on secrecy;[6] in both, she explores the subjects from the perspectives of the individual citizen and of our society and its important institutions. Trust in human relationships depends upon the assumption of
veracity between the participants and trust in societal institutions and in
governments on the part of the people depends upon the perception of
honesty, truth telling, and openness (even assuming the necessity for a
bare minimum of planned secrecy).

At an individual level, she worries that the white lie habit makes it
easier to tell bigger and more significant lies. She thinks the old practices of doctors shielding suffering patients from the truth is now destructive to a proper relationship between doctor and patient. Language
and our speech have brought primacy to the human species and to use
that great gift as the vehicle of deceit is the ultimate perversion. (I wonder if whales or dolphins lie to each other!) Many of the world's leading

philosophers, theologians, and moral leaders have made the point that serious lying is aimed at gaining power over and manipulating other people and is a nonphysical equivalent of doing violence, even at times a kind of murder, to others. M. Scott Peck, the psychiatrist who has also become a best-selling author with his book *The Road Less Travelled*, takes this idea one step further in his more recent treatise, *People of the Lie,*[7] in which he identifies those people who have become rather completely given over to evil as those who lie, essentially continuously, to manipulate others, primarily because they cannot face the truth about themselves.

At a societal or institutional level we seem open to similar criticism: we don't expect the truth from our governments, from our institutions, from our politicians, increasingly from our health professionals, and perhaps most disturbingly from our scientists. A recent major story in *U.S. News and World Report* alleges that cheating in all its forms and at all levels is on the rise in America.[8]

Moreover, several serious scholars recognize in their recent works not only the ubiquity of lying and deceit but their purported importance and value, when used properly, to the health of the individual and of the society as a whole. Walk and Henley present, in essence, views opposed to those of Sissela Bok, referred to earlier.[9] Paul Ekman, in a recently published book, summarizing his researches into accurate recognition of the dissembler by an observer, had this to say,

> Lying is such a central characteristic of life that better understanding of it is relevant to almost all human affairs. Some might shudder at that statement, because they view lying as reprehensible. I do not share that view. It is too simple to hold that no one in any relationship must ever lie; nor would I prescribe that every lie be unmasked.[10]

Ekman quotes George Steiner: "The relevant framework is not one of morality, but of survival. At every level, from brute camouflage to poetic vision, the linguistic capacity to conceal, misinform, leave ambiguous, hypothesize, invent is indispensable to the equilibrium of human consciousness and to the development of man in society."

It is against this societal backdrop that William Broad and Nicholas Wade in their book *Betrayers of the Truth—Fraud and Deceit in the Halls of Science* present a startling analysis of instances of scientific cheating, both in the distant and recent past.[11] They thoughtfully explore the pressures on modern scientists to produce and conform to accepted perceptions of "the truth" and to processes and forms of doing things that often are disincentives to seeking and speaking the truth. They illustrate how easy it is to get supposedly critical people to believe an illusion and, most important, they remind us that the processes of creativity in the "hard" sciences are all of a piece with explorations of the unknown in other creative and scholarly areas.

Science is more than observation and objectivity and the doing of science is more than a constant refinement of observations on nature by new and better techniques. It is also the construction of new models for interpreting nature, of new hypotheses and new paradigms which open up the eyes of the beholder, enabling him or her to see what was always there but simply had escaped recognition.

The point has been made that the "fudging" and manipulation of data by Isaac Newton was of great benefit to society, because otherwise the Newtonian revolution might have been significantly delayed.[12] One could say that such activity by Newton and similarly Einstein falls more into the category of poetic license than scientific fraud. They sought to awaken people to the possibility of a new paradigm whose value could be pragmatically tested and validated or not. Perhaps the need for such "poetic deceptions" would diminish if there were more open-mindedness among scientists. Alternatively and perhaps more logically, one might argue that falsifying data is wrong no matter who does it and no matter what the circumstances and that, in the cases of Newton and Einstein, we choose to ignore these blemishes in the light of their overall performances.

Another element affecting the nature and frequency of dishonesty in the doing of science relates to the fact that there are many sides to "science." Jeremy Bernstein has described Marvin Minsky's work on artificial intelligence; even the uninformed can grasp from his description that a silicon chip with a dramatic new program will either work or it won't—making up data along the way will soon be found out.[13] Similarly, physical chemists and mathematicians cannot frequently lie in their publications without being rapidly uncovered. But biology and biomedical investigations are another matter; the experimental systems are often so complex and so difficult to control adequately that conflicting results are often tolerated for long periods of time. Alternatively, adding a new element to a widely accepted experimental or clinical situation and reporting the expected results will lead to ready publication and a disinterest in checking by another investigator. Thus, one should perhaps expect a greater number of gross examples of cheating in biomedicine than in the "harder" sciences.

A somewhat more frightening example of the stifling of the truth is brought out in Edith Efron's new book, *The Apocalyptics*.[14] Her thesis, laboriously and painstakingly constructed and defended, deals with the more or less official governmental mind-set that presumes that only man-made products cause cancer, mother nature being pure and guiltless in that regard, and that any evidence of carcinogenesis in any animal at any dose is sufficient to ban a product for human consumption. Whether or not one accepts the author's opinions and conclusions, perhaps the most startling fact is that reviewers and expert commentators favorable to the book apparently refused to be identified for fear that their reputations would be forever tainted and their grants would suddenly disappear. That a government view can, in our society, essentially stifle free exchange of opinion to this degree is sobering and demands our attention.

In an interesting cross-cultural analysis of scientific fraud in the People's Republic of China, Richard Suttmeier explores the impact of shifting societal norms on the behavior of scientists in the hope that China's recent experience with apparently increasing corruption will help to distinguish the principal causes of such dishonesty.[15] On the one hand, there are those who maintain that science is no different from any other social institution, and that the behavior of scientists will reflect the dominant normative structure of the whole society. Alternatively, many people believe science is a self-governing institution, marching to its own special drummer and inducing behavior unusually resistant to corrupt practices. Deviant behavior, according to those who share this second view, is strictly an aberrant episode of individual venality.

Suttmeier concludes from his analysis first that "The Chinese case thus seems to support those who claim that corruption in science simply mirrors the patterns of corruption in society." However, he promptly qualifies that conclusion by observing that Chinese science has been bereft of an independent set of normative standards for several decades and that, as a result, Chinese scientists are quite ambiguous about their values. Self-policing in any profession requires clear and unambiguous sets of precepts and shared principles. In the modern western world, it is Robert K. Merton who has made the clearest and most widely accepted statement of norms for the scientific community.[16] These norms, briefly, are as follows: (1) scientists are expected to share the results of their labor; (2) scientists are expected to be critical of the research findings of others and should test them in the laboratory; (3) scientific truths and claims should be true everywhere; and (4) scientific researches should be conducted without regard for material gain or for reputation.

Suttmeier's view seems to be that both the systemic causes of scientific fraud (such as those Broad and Wade described) and the individual aberration are important to the overall understanding of corruption in modern science. If one accepts this view, then one concludes that efforts to improve the situation must include attempts to improve the systemic factors as well as efforts to shore up the individual's moral strength and commitment; and the latter implies the development of a clear and meaningful set of beliefs and normative values for the enterprise.

Since scientific publication has come to play such an important part in the very fabric of modern science and therefore in corrupt practice as well, it might be useful to examine the situation that obtained when scientific journalism began. When Charles II initiated the Royal Society in 1662, he gave life to an international network of scientists linked to the London group through the connections, interest, and hard work of a little-known German, Henry Oldenburg, who had become secretary of the society. Oldenburg's knowledge of languages made him a custommade scientific communications focal point and transmitter. Initially, he communicated through letters from London to the nation and the world. I quote historian Daniel Boorstin on this point in history.

> The letter, which remained for centuries the most "swift, certain, cheap" vehicle of long-distance communication, also expressed a new attitude toward science and new hopes for technology. A letter was suited to communicate a fact or cluster of facts. It signaled an incremental rather than a cosmic approach to experience. The printed scientific "paper" or "article," which was simply a later version of the letter, would be the typical format in which modern science was accumulated and communicated. This form, and the attitude that led scientists to be engrossed with it, declared the appearance of the experimental scientists, in place of the "natural philosopher." The letter was an ideal vehicle for the increasing numbers of men dispersed over Europe who no longer expected to storm the citadel of truth, but hoped to advance knowledge piece by piece.[17]

Oldenburg became, in effect, the originator of scientific journalism and initiated a new era in science when he published in March 1665 the first issue of *Philosophical Transactions*. Let us turn once again to Daniel Boorstin:

> From its very beginnings, Oldenburg's *Phil. Trans.* (as it was familiarly known) had a grand purpose. As he declared in his Introduction to Number 1:
>
> Whereas there is nothing more necessary for promoting the improvement of philosophical Matters, than the communicating to

such, as apply their Studies and Endeavours that way, such things as are discovered or put in practice by others; It is therefore thought fit to employ the *Press,* as the most proper way to gratifie those, whose engagement in such Studies, and delight in the advancement of Learning and profitable Discoveries, doth entitle them to the knowledge of what this Kingdom, or other parts of the World, so, from time to time, afford, as well of the Progress of the Studies, Labors and attempts of the Curious and Learned in things of this kind, as of their complete Discoveries and Performances. To the end, that such Productions being clearly and truly communicated, desires after solide and useful knowledge may be further entertained, ingenious Endeavours and Undertakings cherished, and invited and encouraged to search, try, and find out new things, impart their knowledge to one another, and contribute what they can to the Grand Design of improving Natural knowledge, and perfecting all Philosophical Arts, and Sciences. All for the Glory of God, the Honor and Advantage of these Kingdoms, and the Universal Good of Mankind.

The publication of this first scientific journal was interrupted only twice during Oldenburg's lifetime—once briefly by the plague when the issues came from Oxford instead of London, and then when Oldenburg was put in the Tower of London for his few ill-considered words.

While the *Philosophical Transactions* realized Oldenburg's hopes in ways he could never have imagined, the money rewards were meager. Each monthly issue of about twenty pages printed in twelve hundred copies returned little more than the cost. The enterprise, as Oldenburg's dedication to the society showed, was very much his own, and not until the mid-eighteenth century was publication officially assumed by the society. The *Phil. Trans.* became a model for modern scientific publications. "If all the books in the world except the *Philosophical Transactions* were destroyed," Thomas Henry Huxley observed in 1866, "it is safe to say that the foundations of physical science would remain unshaken, and that the vast intellectual progress of the last two centuries would be largely, though incompletely, recorded."[18]

And thus there began the powerful force of publication in modern science, a force which in itself has become a target for manipulation by those not committed to Oldenburg's high ideals or to those enunciated by Robert Merton. In a certain way, it is correct to say that a scientific discovery does not exist until it is published and thus it becomes crucial for the publication to provide an accurate rendition of the experimentation and results. The motives and rewards of the contributors to Oldenburg's journal have clearly been modified by the external environment for modern scientists.

Jacob Bronowski, the famous physicist-philosopher, believed that free inquiry by the unfettered mind is crucial to the sustenance of a free society.[19] Absolute honesty and commitment to truth telling and truth seeking are the keystones to sustaining free inquiry in a free society, to maintaining fruitful and creative science—and, one assumes, to moving the human race forward on a constructive and positive course in the years ahead. Truth telling is a commitment of each person; each of us can improve or regress in our belief in this regard; and it follows that how well or poorly we do each day is up to each individual and to the general environment established by our society.

Annually, at commencement ceremonies, an army of newly minted young scholars goes forth to conquer the unknown, armed with the tools of a superior education, enormous ambition, and an absolute commitment to truth seeking and truth telling. Everyone in the army seeks to be the first one over the hill and into the enemy camps of ignorance, but they must rely on the commitment to honesty and integrity to temper their ambition and desire to discover new and exciting things. It must be a bit like Socrates' drinking of the hemlock when one of them withholds publication pending a rechecking of a key experiment only to be beaten into print by someone else who started down the track later and might possibly have been a little less careful. Barbara McClintock must have drunk figuratively of Socrates' cup for many years as she tended her garden of corn outside the fancy gene-splicing laboratories in Cold Spring Harbor, New York, under the bemused and somewhat scoffing eyes of more "modern" biologists. But most scientists will not have her ultimate victory and vindication and like Socrates will never know where what they have done finally stands in the scheme of things. Some of them may yield to temptation and conclude that it is better to cheat a little or even a lot and gain increased recognition, honor, or financial reward in the short term; but most of them, we hope, will play it straight and in so doing will protect their profession and their society. They will understand that of the three critical elements of competence, ambition, and integrity, for true scientists the greatest is integrity, for without it scientists will not know their limitations and will contribute to a loss of trust in science and scientists by the society which nurtures it and them.

In closing, let me share the words of Timothy S. Healy, president of Georgetown University, who recently spoke of the great virtues of a university that should not be cast aside.

The first of these is love of truth, the secular, and not always only secular, equivalent of faith. To tell the truth day in and day out, stubbornly, even when it is not popular, is the very base of our community as a university. I pray that Georgetown will never lack men and women whose probity and love of truth can be transmitted to the young in such a way that when in turn their time of temptation or of suffering comes, the memory of it will put steel in their souls and hold them to the truth even if all the world comes tumbling down about their ears.[20]

I cannot escape the conclusion that it requires conscious work and moral effort to maintain honesty throughout one's entire scientific life. It wasn't long ago, in America, that there were no courses in human values or ethics in medical schools; it was assumed that those things were a personal responsibility. Now virtually every school has formal and informal programs and value analysis is extending into continuing medical education. I believe a similar effort should be made in the graduate education of scientists—explorations of a host of issues and circumstances should be undertaken with professional philosophers, ethicists, historians, and social critics. Such education can heighten sensitivities to and understanding of such important matters as relating the structure and organization of science as an institution to the normative values of the scientists and their relative success in minimizing corruption.

The observation has been made that in biomedicine most of the recent examples of fraud and deceit have been perpetrated by M.D.s rather than Ph.D.s.[21] Furthermore, in a recently published study 58 percent of students admitted to cheating during medical school.[22] The implications of these observations are (1) that medical school selects out such ambitious, goal-oriented people that dishonesty is more often selected by them as a pathway to success; and (2) that compared to the medical curriculum, the educational process for Ph.D.s is such as to discourage dishonesty in science. Although both implications may be at least partly true, further studies should be pursued to elucidate these points.

It must not have been easy for Socrates to yield his life and drink the hemlock; and it is interesting to speculate on the impact of his life and work on subsequent generations had he not done so. A lifetime of commitment, analysis, and discussion prepared him for his time of trial and it is reasonable to assume that scientists in training and in practice can similarly profit from ongoing considerations of the key ethical issues of their trade, the most basic of which are related to honesty, integrity, truth seeking, and truth speaking.

One hopes that no scientist would need to drink figuratively from the Socratic cup of hemlock, but my most fervent wish is that all would be willing to do so rather than compromise the truth. Experience tells me that many, if not all of them, in fact, will have to sip at least nonlethal quantities from that bitter cup from time to time in order to keep their integrity and preserve the honor of their profession.

Let me summarize my own perceptions and opinions on these matters. Science as a social institution is value-based. Truth telling and truth seeking are the essential and fundamental values undergirding the trust of our society in the modern scientific enterprise. There is evidence that these values are being compromised (if they are in fact not crumbling) as basic cornerstones of our society and that more and more examples of such transgressions against the truth are being noted in science. It is relatively easy to commit fraud or to deceive colleagues and the public in the biomedical sciences; the incentives to publish at almost any cost are great. Money, power, and advancement all play major roles in affecting the individual scientist operating within a society which has deified competition as a process and winning as a goal.

Regardless of whether or not historians will one day determine whether what we are observing is only a minor trend as against a major tide and dramatic shift in direction, it behooves us to treat the situation as serious. To do so requires action at the societal and institutional levels, such as developing educational initiatives and alterations of incentives to untruthful behavior, and action by individual scientists, each of whom must realize that to be honest day in and day out inevitably will require sacrifice. The scientist should in my view be able to accept and incorporate that sacrifice meaningfully into his or her world view in order to sustain a sense of satisfaction throughout a lifetime of scientific investigation.

If the critical mass of our institutions and of our scientists so orient themselves, we shall preserve our values of truth telling and truth seeking and thus preserve the societal trust in science so essential for continued discovery and progress. In so doing, perhaps the scientific and academic communities can show the way to the rest of the society.

## Notes

1. Evelyn Fox Keller, *A Feeling for the Organism—The Life and Work of Barbara McClintock* (New York: W. H. Freeman and Co., 1983), 3–13.

2. Karl Jaspers, *Socrates, Buddha, Confucius, Jesus, a Harvest* (New York and London: Harcourt Brace Jovanovich, 1962).

3. Karl Lamb, *The Guardians—Leadership Values and the American Tradition* (New York: W. W. Norton, 1982).

4. Roger Bulger, "Notes of a Lewis Thomas Watcher: Emerging Intellectual Unities," *Pharos* 47 (Spring 1984): 25–26.

5. Sissela Bok, *Lying—Moral Choice in Public and Private Life* (New York: Random House, 1979).

6. Sissela Bok, *Secrets—On the Ethics of Concealment and Revelation* (New York: Pantheon Books, 1982).

7. M. Scott Peck, *People of the Lie—The Hope for Healing Human Evil* (New York: Simon and Schuster, 1983).

8. "Why Cheating Is on the Rise in the U.S.," *U.S. News and World Report*, March 5, 1984, 53–54.

9. Robert L. Walk and Arthur Henley, *The Right to Lie: A Psychological Guide to the Uses of Deceit in Everyday Life* (New York: Peter H. Wyden, 1970).

10. Paul Ekman, *Telling Lies—Clues to Deceit in the Marketplace, Politics and Marriage* (New York and London: W. W. Norton, 1985), 23.

11. William Broad and Nicholas Wade, *Betrayers of the Truth—Fraud and Deceit in the Halls of Science* (New York: Simon and Schuster, 1983).

12. Laurence Tancredi, personal communication.

13. Jeremy Bernstein, *Science Observed* (New York: Basic Books, 1982), 9–121.

14. Edith Efron, *The Apocalyptics, Cancer and the Big Lie, How Environmental Politics Controls What We Know about Cancer* (New York: Simon and Schuster, 1984).

15. Richard P. Suttmeier, "Corruption in Science: The Chinese Case," *Science, Technology and Human Values* 10 (Winter 1985): 49–61.

16. Robert K. Merton, ed., *The Sociology of Science* (Chicago: University of Chicago Press, 1973).

17. Daniel J. Boorstin, *The Discoverers* (New York: Random House, 1983), 391.

18. Ibid., 393.

19. Jacob Bronowski, *A Sense of the Future* (Cambridge, Mass.: MIT Press, 1977).

20. Timothy S. Healy, "The Doing of Truth," in *Georgetown University 1983 Annual Report* (Washington, D.C., 1984).

21. Robert K. Kuttner, "Fraud in Science," *Science* 227, no. 4686 (February 1985): 466.

22. F. Sierles, I. Hendricks, and S. Circle, "Cheating in Medical School," *Journal of Medical Education* 55 (1980): 124–125.

# 8. *Emerging Unities of the Twenty-first Century: Service as Sacrament, Emotional Neutrality, and the Power of the Therapeutic Word*

Roger J. Bulger

Consider the twenty-first century and what it will bring to the profession of medicine. Surely, no one is qualified to speak to the next century, even if one limits one's target to a consideration of medical ethics and the nature of the profession of medicine, because such a target inevitably reaches to the philosophy and nature of the entire society. No one is qualified to address these questions with certainty and confidence; therefore, anyone may address them if he or she does so with the proper perspective and humility. Of course, a trained social scientist, philosopher, theologian, or a practicing poet, prophet, or seer would each bring some particular strength to such a discussion of the future. I write hopefully as an intelligent, reasonably well-educated, and concerned citizen; as someone interested in the universe in which he lives; as someone concerned about the society of humans of which he is a part and how those humans go about conducting their business; as someone committed to an optimism about the future of the evolutionary progress of the world and its inhabitants; and as someone involved with most others in the seem-

ingly never ending quest for individual meaning and purpose. Having
stated those biases, it is perhaps acceptable for me to take your time
with my musings on these matters.

There is an old Zen Buddhist saying which goes,

> Those who know, do not speak;
> Those who speak, do not know!

A friend of mine has another favorite saying that fits this and many
other moments: "The only time a whale can get harpooned is when he
rises to the surface to spout off." With all these caveats, it is nevertheless important for us to discuss these matters as best we can among
ourselves.

I believe that the discoveries and insights of the past twenty-five years
have brought about a variety of what I shall refer to as emerging intellectual unities. Increasingly, it seems that in several important areas
there are tendencies to an intellectual unification of previously unrelated
or even heretofore mutually exclusive ideas. I would like to discuss three
such areas which may not be connected to one another by any compelling logic but which are associated in my own mind. The first area has
to do with the growing together of science and the arts, including philosophy and theology; the second with the centrality of language to the
development of the human species as perceived by philosophers and
rhetoricians on the one hand and by scientists on the other; and the third
with the merging of the science and art of medicine in the attempt to
achieve a therapeutic relationship in the practice of medicine.

Einstein's friend and colleague Max Born, a Nobelist in theoretical
physics, said that "Physics is philosophy," and he meant it. Jacob
Bronowski, noted scientist and author of *The Ascent of Man,* desired
to create a modern philosophy that would bring science and humanity
together in a single conceptual piece. He believed that all science is philosophy but that without humanity there could be neither a decent philosophy nor a decent science. For Bronowski, a person became creative,
as an artist or as a scientist, when he or she uncovered a new unity in
the variety of nature. Bronowski discerned a unity of nature which made
nature's laws seem beautiful in their simplicity. Whether he succeeded or
not in creating a compelling new modern philosophy for the twentieth
century, Bronowski did succeed in illustrating repeatedly the unity of
the creative act in science and the arts.

For the public, especially the increasing numbers of well-educated
lay people, the explosive expansions of new knowledge over the past
quarter-century have had a startling effect on philosophic and even the-
ologic considerations and have made efforts like Bronowski's toward a

unitary philosophy seem possible of attainment. As a college student in
the fifties it seemed to me that the weight of "scientific evidence" told
us first, that our evolution from our primate ancestors and ultimately
from the primordial slime was a result of a series of random biological
events which took place between two ice ages and that our future would
be as a frozen relic in a small corner of the universe, by then completely
abandoned; second, that the molecular biologists, when they had un-
locked the riddles of DNA, would have solved the last of biology's important mysteries and that even the biochemistry of a thought would soon
be ready for molecular dissection; third, that the atom had been smashed,
fully understood down to its basics, reassembled, and "harnessed" and
that was that in atomic physics; fourth, that Einstein and the modern astronomers had settled the questions about the universe, which was infinitely expanding; and fifth, that our earth had limited resources which
human greed, ignorance, and lust would exhaust within a few hundred
years. There was little room for the searching, informed lay person of
twenty-five years ago to keep these items side by side with a traditional
religious cosmology; and there was a feeling among the religious, the
poets, philosophers, and artists that science was fearful, that the search
for new facts and new technologies was threatening to established values, philosophies, and even theologies.

But all that seems to have changed, and the dawning in the public
mind of this change has been coincident with the emergence of Dr.
Lewis Thomas as one of the most articulate spokespeople in the English
language of the new lessons of the biological sciences.

His messages are several, often repeated in his writing, and they may
be found hidden in the interstices between his parablelike expositions of
this or that particular piece of nature's fabric. Whether he is explaining
the life cycle of the mimosa girdler or wondering over the fantastic coordination of the society of the weaver ant, he always comes back, explicitly or by indirection, to his belief that the human race is not a dead end,
that the special human trait is the capacity to learn and that searching
for truth is the only way that we can work out our future with all its extraordinary problems.

Recalling that Socrates taught that fools think they are wise while
the wise know that they are fools and remembering how central to the
whole Socratic approach this important theme was, let us consider
Lewis Thomas' view of the magnificent contributions of science: "The
greatest single achievement of science in this most scientifically productive of centuries is the discovery that we are profoundly ignorant: We
know very little about nature and we understand even less."[1]

Thomas' emphasis on what we do not know has helped to bring into
perspective for the public the remaining great mysteries of the universe;

this perspective has been underscored by the growing public awareness of the transience of particular scientific theories, a transience that has been demonstrated many times within the lifetimes of most of us. The atom is now more than electrons, protons, and neutrons; the universe has black holes and maybe even boundaries; the exploration of space makes possible the conceptualization of a life after earth for whatever the human race may have become by then; the revelations of the molecular biologist are recognized as rather primitive discoveries foreshadowing much, much more rather than representing a final understanding of an ultimate biological reality; the computer revolution, only at its inception, offers the literal promise of almost instantaneous communication throughout the world and the development of a kind of world-consciousness. The Black Hole and the Big Bang sound a lot like the biblical concept of creation and, as the mysteries and the wonderings deepen, the thinking of philosophers and theologians as diverse as Gabriel Marcel and Teilhard de Chardin seem to be converging on a spot shared by the Bronowskis and Thomases of the scientific world. So modern science has expanded our minds and opened up new conceptual possibilities and its supporters see in its products the need and compulsion to keep learning.

Even when Lewis Thomas speaks as a physician to physicians, one can bring his views to a synchrony with thinkers like Marcel. Thomas makes plain how futile was the therapeutic armamentarium available to his father, who served a rural population for years as a general practitioner, but he writes with understanding about the value of the human support and alleviation of pain and mental suffering such compassionate physicians could bring to their patients then and can bring even now.

Dr. Thomas is at the interface between science and humanity—partly because his "science" is biological and in fact has relevance to human health and disease and partly because he is a physician, a leader in that profession most intensively involved in bringing the fruits of science and technology to bear upon the problems of the human condition. He is an important figure in our culture's intellectual life largely because he does bring together in his career and writings the two themes of human service and the optimistic and inexorable human need to keep learning while recognizing the uncertainties and ambiguities of our situation.

It is interesting to reflect on the convergence of these themes with those also expressed by the modern French philosopher Gabriel Marcel in his book *Man against Mass Society:*

> It is precisely in the name of an inward-turned and self-centered conception of equality that people claim the right today to rise in rebellion against the idea of service. In that way, we turn our backs

on the possibility of real fraternity, that is, on every possibility of
humanizing our relations with our fellow men. . . . And here we
come upon an unexpected and yet central aspect of our theme. To
serve, in the valuable senses of the word, implies above all to serve
truth, and perhaps it is by the help of this illumination that we can
best perceive what it is to serve in the absolute sense of the word,
that is to serve God . . .[2]

Lewis Thomas and Jacob Bronowski don't use the word "God"; but if
one substitutes "God" for "truth" in their writings one can clearly see
the overlapping of ideas among them. Granted that Marcel might well
have a richer or more complicated set of descriptors for God than truth,
the point is nevertheless made.

For his part, Thomas allows blind faith to enter in only to his basic
conviction that there must be a purpose for the evolution of the human
being and that *homo sapiens* is not a dead end on the evolutionary path.
This leads him to the following conclusion in one of his recent essays:
"But I think we can make a guess at one kind of answer to my question:
what are human beings good at, really good at as a species, making us
worth all the trouble we cause? For the very long run, learning is what
we are good at, and if we keep at it long enough we may one day begin
to pay our way."[3]

Although it is clear that Teilhard de Chardin is hardly in the mainstream of orthodox Catholic theology, his mysticism, spirituality, and
credentials as both a deeply believing Christian and a practicing scientist seem beyond question, and his influence seems to be growing.
Thomas M. King, in his recently published analysis of Teilhard, observed that Teilhard's essential message is that he experienced God most
profoundly when he was actually doing his science, trying to learn new
things. This represents an example of what is called process theology
which has its advocates and detractors and its conclusion and corollaries;
but Teilhard's meaning sums up what for me may be an important
emerging unity for the next century.

We have come a long way from the time when we believed only what
we saw, smelled, touched, tasted, or heard. The doubting Thomas has
a much harder time these days, because we are measuring and quanti-
fying things that are beyond the limits of human sensing abilities; sub-
microscopic and spectacularly cosmic realities are scientific dogma now
which, years ago, would have been grist for the mystic's mill. Increasingly, direct observations are filtered through computers, analyzed, and
received as a printout by the human observer. If this is so now and is
likely to be more so in the future, let us consider for a few moments

what the implications are of all this for medicine, for Hippocrates' "silent art."

Let me introduce my response to this question by referring once again to Lewis Thomas who, from his perspective as a biologist viewing the evolutionary process, has identified language as the most advanced and distinctive characteristic of our species, holding the key to our further development. Cleanth Brooks, the well-known professor emeritus of rhetoric at Yale University, comes at the primacy of language from a totally different perspective. He sees science as the knowledge of means whereas the arts provide knowledge of the ends; for him, language is the transmitter of human value systems from generation to generation and the study of literature, intellectual history, comparative cultures, and so forth are immersions in human values, in ends. Brooks thus joins forces with I. A. Richards, another famous rhetorician, in believing that language is crucial to the development of civilized culture. Thus, from their varying beginning points, Brooks, Richards, and Thomas (and of course many others) all converge in agreement on the centrality of language for the further evolution of our species.

Where does medicine stand in relation to this primacy of language? Hippocrates and his followers took medicine away from the soothsayers, spell casters, and verbal magicians of previous ages and made the profession active in observation, diagnosis, and treatment. Doctors became doers, people of action, seeking to find new and better methods of intervening in disease processes. Medicine became the silent art. In fact, however, there wasn't all that much scientific to either remain silent about or to talk about until the past half-century, when truly effective technologies have been tumbling from science laboratories and industrial development efforts in an ever-increasing cascade.

Prior to this time of technological and specialty proliferation, much of what the doctor really had to offer was human support. The public supposedly longs for the old days when such human support was apparently in such abundant supply, but most people seem to accept the twenty-first century inevitability that ours is likely to be a depersonalized assembly-line, computer-based medical care system. As we ponder the incredible technological advances of the recent past and the even more astounding prospects for the next two decades and beyond, it is easy to conclude that the dichotomy in medicine begun by Hippocrates' division of the talkers from the doers will at last become complete. Even the stethoscope, the symbol of a direct contact between patient and doctor, is rapidly becoming outmoded. History taking is automated or delegated; much of the physical exam can be handled in similar fashion. Spectacular new noninvasive scanning devices can provide unbelievably detailed analyses of abnormalities without even requiring the patient to speak to a doctor. And so on.

On the surface, then, one may argue that the medicine of the future will be guided by professionals trained in high technology, with little time for, interest in, or skill at the techniques of supporting ill people and their families. Further, one could contend that the "silent art" should remain ever more silent, because it is simply not cost-effective for such expensively educated medical technocrats to indulge in the human support function.

An alternative argument can be made, based in part upon the growing body of scientific evidence connecting the impact of a highly charged word from someone else upon an individual's body biochemistry. It can be more readily appreciated now that what people say to other people can often have an effect for good or ill on the soma. Because of the unprecedented technological power now at our command, the physician, as the kind of high priest of science, is in an extraordinarily advantageous position to benefit or influence the patient even more than previously with his or her words and other forms of human support; with this realization, it then becomes possible to seriously consider an alternative to the current trend toward depersonalized medicine.

It is our purpose here to explore the proposition that in the next century our silent art should be silent no more, that we should divest ourselves of this aspect of our Hippocratic heritage which makes it more difficult for many doctors to become true healers. In order to approach this proposition, consideration shall be given to the nature and concept of service, the quality of emotional involvement in relations with patients, an exploration of the history of the spoken word as a therapeutic tool, and some reflections on the primacy of technical and professional competence as the first rule of medical ethics. It is possible to postulate that the right mixture of competence, commitment to service, and a greater facility with the use of words and other forms of communication in dealing with people can produce the most powerful and humane healing profession the world has ever known.

A special commitment to serving other people is an essential part of the ethos of the profession of medicine and presumably of each of that profession's practicing members. Without it, the profession cannot continue with the public trust and confidence it now enjoys.

This special commitment does not mean that the doctor must work 90 or 120 hours a week; it does not mean that the doctor must suffer a ruination of any or all nonprofessional responsibilities, such as the family or civic or church activities. It simply acts to define the foundation of the relationship when there is an interaction between doctor and patient.

There are a few things this special commitment should not mean or imply. It should not serve to disguise the ego satisfaction and sometimes excessive and unnecessary secondary gain received from happy patients which often makes it more pleasant and appealing for doctors to stay with their patients than return to their more routine family responsibilities. This special commitment should not be construed as the charter for an elite and exclusive club or for the establishment of a false pride. Rather, it establishes the basis for trust and action for any human service profession, whether it be teaching, the ministry, dentistry, social service, or medicine.

Recently, one of medicine's truly great and wise leaders, Walsh McDermott, discussed Samaritanism in medical practice and called for a return to the human support function as a part of the doctor's armamentarium. He used, as a personal example, a situation in the early 1940s when a beautiful young woman was admitted to the hospital with a fulminating case of erysipelas. Her face was swollen, she was almost incoherent, and her temperature was 105°F. A few short years before she might easily have been dead by morning; instead Dr. McDermott gave her penicillin and watched her fever drop and mental state return to normal overnight. When he went to see his handiwork the next morning, he assured the patient the danger was over and acceded to her request for a mirror without a second thought. The sight of her badly reddened and disfigured face absolutely devastated her, she was inconsolable because she believed her looks would never return, and she remained miserable for the several days it took for the inflammation to subside and her face to return to normal.

Dr. McDermott contended that his commitment to serve that patient was not complete and by failing to place her first he had caused her considerable suffering and felt the discomfort of not having performed as a complete physician. He went on to point out that his ambition to become a superior physician soon led him to recognize and emulate those role models he most admired in their attempts to provide human support for their patients. Finally, he stated that such behavior can be learned and produces such wonderful responses from appreciative patients that most doctors will adopt this mode of relating to patients.

In this discussion of Samaritanism according to McDermott, there is much that overlaps with our consideration of a special commitment to serve. Again, Marcel had a great deal to say about the concept of service, the decline of which he linked with the rise of egalitarian societies dedicated to the masses.[4] For Marcel, equality had come to mean that each person is just as good as each other person and owes that other person nothing beyond that which our technocratic and bureaucratic society determines we are to produce for our day's pay. We do that much and no more. Lost, he says, is the sense of loyalty, fidelity, and attachment that the old-time family servant used to exemplify in his or her relations with the family. He asks in a variety of ways, what will become of service in a bureaucratic world? and his question has an unmatched immediacy for modern medicine.

Marcel made much of this concept of service because he saw in its demise the ultimate destruction of civilized society. He believed that individuals cannot be or remain free without a linkage to that which transcends them, and he saw the key expression of that linkage through the old idea of service to others. His ideas have a further relevance to us in that he attaches a special importance to the notion of service to the poor, weak, and sick: "I think I should be formulating my thoughts fairly exactly if I said that each of us has a duty to multiply as much as possible around him the bonds between being and being. . . . Fraternity is centered on the other person. . . . It is just as if one's consciousness projected itself towards the other person, towards my neighbor . . ."[5]

Marcel's ideas lend themselves easily to parallel considerations regarding the nature of the doctor-patient relationship. First, doctors serve their family of patients much as traditional house servants loyally served the family in whose home they resided—with "attachment and fidelity."

Second, at its best the nature of the interaction must be based on the complete certainty that doctors are participating in this interaction fundamentally to benefit patients. True, a living can be earned, but doctors are not primarily gaining money, power, influence, or any other favors or advantages from patients; they are not becoming famous through experimentation at patients' expense. They are there to be of help to a diseased fellow human being, and it is the purity and intensity of that motivation which if accurately communicated to patients allows them to relax in confidence and have a better chance of healing themselves. Third, fidelity to the patient goes hand in hand with fidelity to the truth.

Surely this simple commitment describes the ideal for the teacher-student interaction as well as nurse or dentist or speech therapist/patient-client interaction. Surely the commitment is unusual and could be accused of promoting elitism, but I would argue the true healers are an elite group.

The commitment to the patient must be genuine and it is not always felt equally strongly at all times toward all patients, so it requires conscious and consistent labor of the will. It seems as though we are discussing, as Professor Stanley Hauerwas says, a kind of training of oneself in virtue, and indeed we are, but no more than any other workers should train themselves to excellence in their work. However, it is true that for a healing relationship to endure or obtain even transiently it is our thesis that the patient must trust the doctor's commitment. In fact, it is the aggregate of each patient's feelings about his or her doctor in this regard that forms the basis for the aggregate public image of the medical profession.

Philosophical and religious overtones notwithstanding, we speak here only of what goes on ideally between doctor and patient in the treating mode. The doctor, off work, may operate however he or she sees fit, of course, so we are not demanding overall sanctity. Like the athletic virtuoso—poetry in motion on the court or field but hard drinking and high living off the court—there is no *a priori* requirement that the doctor behave in certain ways outside the relationship with patients. The demands of social pressure and patient expectations have, however, for centuries dictated a fairly high degree of conformity to the highest standards of social behavior for physicians. It is important here to emphasize that what is described here is what I believe to be an essential component for the achievement of an optimal environment in which the patient can best do his or her part in the healing process.

The question of the proper emotional stance for the doctor vis-à-vis the patient is not a simple one. The one "rule" that relates to the need for a certain emotional detachment from the patient states that doctors should not treat members of their own families, and even this dictum is not rigidly adhered to. Most people believe that doctors should be sympathetic toward their patients. Sometimes empathy is the word used to describe the desired trait.

I have always had trouble with those two words (sympathy and empathy) as they relate to the doctor-patient relationship, partly because it is not possible to sympathize with each person on purely emotional grounds. The Webster International Unabridged Dictionary defines empathy as "the capacity for participating in or a vicarious experiencing of another's feelings, volitions, or ideas and sometimes another's movements to the point of executing bodily movements resembling his." Sympathy is a synonym for empathy as defined above, but Webster comes closer to what we seek in a doctor with a second definition, as follows, "the act or capacity of entering into or sharing the feelings or interests of another—the character or fact of being sensitive to or affected by another's emotions, experiences or especially sorrows."

No one has enough emotional energy to be affected by a patient's situation in ways similar to the patient's own reactions. To feel grief every time a patient feels grief, anxiety every time a patient feels anxiety, and so on is folly, and to attempt to reach such a stage is equally foolish. On the other hand, I should say I have been scolded several times regarding this point; some people believe it is good to cry with the patient, at least at times. Although I can conceive of situations when it is not a negative event to emote side by side with the patient, it is my belief that such events are in general not good for the healing relationship.

Sympathy and empathy are inadequate to describe the quality we need. Perhaps there needs to be a new word to describe the capacity to appreciate and understand the feelings and mental state of another and to convey support and strength while remaining personally separate from the other's condition. The prefix *eu* connotes working toward positive outcomes and therefore perhaps "eupathy" is the word we should create to describe the stance of the doctor toward the suffering person.

The finest literary example of eupathy of which I am aware may be found in T. S. Eliot's play *The Confidential Clerk*. The main character is open and truthful but seems detached, indifferent, and uninvolved with each of the other characters, each of whom benefits through a kind of healing relationship with this seemingly distant person. In one way or another each of the other characters tries to capture his emotions, but ultimately they all agree that he should have no emotionally binding entanglements—that his being detached and uninvolved regarding his own interests is essential for him to fill his role. In fact, the main character's speech, demeanor, and behavior are all exemplary, illustrating concern, a sense of responsibility, competence, and a desire to serve efficiently, warmly, and compassionately. In effect, he encourages those he knows to know themselves better, to fulfill their own potentialities more completely, and to work out their own destinies and healings.

Eliot's character may be translatable into the dynamics of the healing medical relationship in that it is possible to achieve a sensitivity to each patient's status and to combine that with a communicated support for improvement. Emotional neutrality may not be the best word to approximate eupathy, but it comes closer to what we need than does sympathy or empathy and is equally compatible with the adoption of a friendly demeanor.

Among the several continuing threads of the history of western medicine is one concerning the place of the word in therapy or, put another way, of speech in the contextual relationship between patient and physician. I predict that the therapeutic value of the word, particularly as it relates to the speech of the physician, will be increasingly respected by clinicians in the years ahead. Further, I believe that the dynamics of the therapeutic relationship should continue to be the subject of systematic study and analysis and that motivated, intelligent students can learn how to use speech as a therapeutic tool and avoid its adverse reactions and sometimes all-too-toxic effects.

As scholars of linguistics point out, early human society relied almost solely on speech to communicate. Even in ancient Greece, after the introduction of the written word, the great orators remained the most influential of people; the rhetorician was also the philosopher and was supposed to be the repository of all knowledge.

As writing and symbolic thinking in mathematics came to the fore, the primacy of speech was threatened and ultimately lost. Pedro Lain Entralgo, a Spanish psychiatrist and classical Greek scholar, in his book *The Therapy of the Word in Classical Antiquity,* outlines clearly the role of therapeutic speech in Greek culture, although in his view the word never became a therapeutic tool until Freud developed modern psychotherapy in the late nineteenth and early twentieth centuries.

A thousand years before Plato, Homer wrote of three different uses of the word to benefit the sick: cheering speech, wherein the speaker encourages the diseased person and offers human support; prayers to gods beseeching their intervention on behalf of the sufferer; and magic incantations or spells which a shaman of one sort or another utilizes to cure the patient. Plato recognized the word as a therapeutic tool as described above and allowed it a place in his Republic, but he specifically excluded the poets and playwrights from his ideal kingdom because those writers' words excited passions in the listener, which to Plato could lead to no good end.

For Lain Entralgo, this recognition by Plato of the emotion-stirring qualities of drama and poetry established the foundation for the psychotherapeutic intervention. Aristotle explicated the value of an emotional catharsis, which people can experience by watching a play, and he believed that such releases of pent-up emotion were highly desirable and therapeutic. Lain Entralgo claims that Aristotle's treatment of poetry and the arts was sufficiently complete that the Greeks at that point had all the intellectual substratum required to create the new field of psychotherapy. Why, then, didn't it happen?

Surprisingly, the culprits seem to have been Hippocrates and his followers. Hippocrates, as we all know, emphasized careful observation and, where appropriate, specific physical intervention to cure the patient's ills. He regarded with great disfavor those who cast charms over diseases with their words; the tradition of using words to treat the sick was at cross purposes with the budding science of medicine. The Hippocratic corpus continued this trend, in effect for centuries institutionalizing medicine as "the silent art," an art based on nature, observation, reasoning, and action.

Admittedly, the writings of Hippocrates and his followers are replete with explicit advice and implications regarding moral behavior, confidentiality, and even occasionally what may be considered sensitive ways to treat patients which include decorous and appealing habits of speech. The essential thrust was clear, however: talk cures nothing and this great art of medicine is basically silent.

As recently as fifty years ago, western physicians had little in the way of effective technological intervention to offer patients. What tools they did have usually didn't work or were downright harmful. The idealized doctors of that age, now often envisioned as committed humanitarians whose practice site was the patient's home, had in fact mostly words to offer to ameliorate suffering. They offered human support; they would personally stand by the patient and advise the family as they watched their patients through an illness.

In the 1980s, with such wonderfully effective new tools in our possession, many doctors think we don't need to do that sort of thing. Our first obligation is to maintain competence—an awesome responsibility these days—and that means a continuing investment in science and technology. We need to be expert in those interventions we now have at our disposal which are so effective in treating diseases or symptoms. According to our education, X-rays, hormones, chemotherapy, antidepressants, analgesics, and CAT scans are highly effective tools; words are not. We are all too often uncomfortable with words, embarrassed by or ineffectual with them, and we see them as without value in the fight against a tangible disease. We are more than ever embedded in the silent art.

Why is all of this somehow disquieting? In part, we are disquieted because as the profession seems to be ever more effective in utilizing its science and technology, the public is increasingly critical and disaffected. We are accused of being inhumane, mechanistically oriented, and materialistic. Although most doctors realize at some level that their words can have tremendous impact, at least on some patients, it's just not a scientific thing. Most doctors have never thought, nor do they think now, of words as a mode of therapy.

Against this background science is once again leading us to some new concepts which may produce a rationale through which most doctors could come to consider their speech as therapeutically significant. Among the modern advances in neurochemistry there are many observations relating the emotional state to the production of certain chemicals or secretion of certain hormones. For example, the endorphins of the brain are endogenous morphinelike substances, the production or secretion of which may in fact be influenced by a variety of external influences. It thus becomes an easy thing to envision how the doctor could use words as therapy if he or she only knew how to affect the patient's emotional state in an appropriate manner.

There are many examples of such interventions and I'm certain every superior physician has several from his or her own experience. One of the purest illustrations is referred to by Norman Cousins in his book *The Anatomy of an Illness* when he quotes Bernie Lown, the noted Harvard cardiologist, on his treatment of a patient with an acute myocardial infarction.[6] According to Dr. Lown, the most important therapeutic beginning can be for the doctor to meet his or her recently stricken heart patient in the emergency room and tell the patient that everything is under control and that he or she will be all right. Dr. Lown seldom has to give the traditional shot of morphine to these patients and an important initial step toward recovery has been taken. In this instance it is clear that the word and the trust relationship have been used as therapy.

Many studies on the placebo effect have suggested that information extended through the trust relationship of patient and physician has lessened perceived pain and reduced requirements for analgesic medications. Most thoughtful physicians can remember instances when they wished that words spoken could be gotten back, just as they can remember when they wished they could have back a drug or operation that produced an unfortunate side effect.

The observation that western medicine, beginning in the fifth century B.C. with Hippocrates, associated itself with action rather than words may explain what could otherwise be construed as a most peculiar and persistent separation of medicine from the great healers and healing associated with religion and religious leaders. The power of belief, whether it be in touching the prophet, going to Lourdes, or accepting Christian Science, is obviously a most powerful therapeutic tool. Although one explanation for these phenomena may be a pure and simple divine intervention external to the patient, another may be related to the impact on the disease of an altered mental status and belief structure on the part of the patient. We tend to think of these healers and "miraculous" cures as being in the past from the prescientific medical era, but, in fairness, even the most skeptical among us must recognize that these things continue to occur among the simple and the sophisticated, affecting people with access to all the high technology that modern medicine has to offer. Not only have we no explanation, but modern science has done little to pursue possible explanations for these phenomena.

Anyone who has ever sacrificed experimental rats by exposure to ether in a jar knows how some fight the anesthetic far more vigorously than others. Apparently there is some evidence that patients who get angry at having cancer fight it more effectively than do those more passive souls who seem more willing to accept death.

All these observations tend to support the view that one aim of the therapeutic relationship should be for physicians to aid patients to attain a state of mind in which patients most optimally may cure themselves or aid the external technical interventions in the curative process. To do this requires a lot more knowledge and a lot more insight, understanding, and analysis of what makes some patients get well and others not and of how the doctor can influence the process by his or her behavior and speech.

What is this therapy of the word? I have included Homer's cheering speech (which sounds like an ancient equivalent of a good bedside manner), followed Lain Entralgo's arguments about psychotherapy as word or logo-therapy, and implicated all the human support functions arising from a successful doctor-patient relationship through a consideration of Walsh McDermott's idea of medical Samaritanism and the example of Dr. Lown's approach to a patient with myocardial infarction. Finally, I have touched upon the religious or faith healers and implied that there may be some important linkages between them and traditional medicine.

I do not mean to imply by this analysis that the physician should acquire the techniques of the faith healer or aspire to produce miracles out of the power of his or her words or personality. Rather, I argued that the combination of the tremendous power of modern science and medical technology resting in the physician's hands and the frightening abyss traversed by those afflicted by a major disease create the environment out of which various levels of a healing relationship can be established. The sensitive and motivated physician can work at his or her role throughout a lifetime of practice and from time to time for some patients be the instrument through which a real cure emerges by virtue of a relationship that will be beneficial to both patient and doctor. Scientific physician-healers must remain firmly rooted in their science but they may be able to learn to tap some of the emotional reserves seemingly open to nontraditional healers. Therein lies a challenge which should be taken up.

In the ancient oral cultures, spoken words had an enormous power and immediacy difficult for moderns to appreciate. The power which primitive people attached to spoken words through charms and spells and which Hippocrates and his followers down through the present time have ascribed to magic or to religious faith may in fact have some intelligible biochemical explanation. Today, as Professor Walter Ong says: ". . . the world moves in the new orality of our electronic era, where the telephone, loudspeaker, radio and television give voice a new kind of currency. Our new secondary orality makes us in significant ways like those who lived in the old primary oral culture . . ."[7]

One wonders, as our physical exams become more cursory and physical touching of the patient becomes less prominent, if the verbal interchange will not become even more important. Medicine is ready for a new look at the use of the word in treatment. The subject needs exploration and analysis; it needs to be expanded conceptually beyond classical psychotherapy; it needs emphasis and to be taught wherever it can be.

I believe such study has begun and that an emerging unity in medical practice is becoming clearer, a partial reunification of the old mind/body duality, which will be recognized one day as one of the great contributions of the twenty-first century.

The last words in this essay should deal briefly with some of Ed Pellegrino's ideas. Pellegrino has for years placed medicine squarely at the intersection of philosophy and science and believes medicine is a kind of "cutting edge" social institution capable of enriching both the arts and the sciences. With this theme he shares his interests with Bronowski and Thomas.

Perhaps more important in the long run for the profession of medicine is Pellegrino's definition of the physician's role and his analysis of the patient-physician relationship. Pellegrino emphasizes the fact that there are now at least a half-dozen different theories and models of medicine, each of which, if followed, leads to its own implications for medical practice for health-related public policy. He systematically rejects most of them, including the purely biomedical model recently advocated by Seldin and the health promotion approach of Leon Kass.

For Pellegrino, medicine is defined as a healing relationship with the goal of reaching a particular decision at a particular time which is both right and good for the patient. He sees medicine as a moral enterprise scientifically based. Thus the "right" decision is scientifically correct; the "good" decision is one which fits in best with the patient's being and circumstances. The doctor says to the patient, "I have knowledge and I shall put it to use in your best interest according to your direction." The doctor's primary moral responsibility to his or her patients is the sustaining of technical competence. Pellegrino defines compassion as that capacity of the doctor to place the right decision inside the patient's circumstances such that it will be good for the patient. Thus, Pellegrino comes to a view of medicine which remains intensely personal and practical, in which the sciences and the arts are brought together at specific instances where specific decisions must be reached by two people acting in concert, the patient and the doctor, pilgrims in search of a cure. Perhaps that's the proper image on which to conclude my discussion of emerging unities of the next century—the twenty-first century unity of patient and doctor searching together for a better future for the patient.

## Notes

1. L. Thomas, "How Should Humans Pay Their Way?" *New York Times,* August 24, 1981, 19.

2. G. Marcel, *Man against Mass Society* (Chicago: Henry Regnery Co., 1962), 208–209.

3. Thomas, "How Should Humans," 19.

4. Marcel, *Man against Mass Society*.

5. Ibid.

6. N. Cousins, *Anatomy of an Illness* (New York: W. W. Norton, 1979).

7. W. Ong, *The Therapy of the Word in Classical Antiquity* (New Haven: Yale University Press, 1970).

# PART III.

*The Healing Context:*
*Cultures, Persons, and Words*

# 9. *The Anthropology of Healing*

**Lola Romanucci-Ross
and Laurence R. Tancredi**

Physicians have practiced their art within a framework of high moral sensitivity.[1] This moral sensitivity is based on a code of ethics as well as on tacit expectations of the physician's role, both of which have evolved over the centuries.[2] Moral codes and physician roles are field dependent on a more basic structure that defines how human beings should function with and relate to other human beings, particularly where a special duty or relationship exists. All of these phenomena exist within the cultural context.

Similarly, medical systems involving the physician, other health care providers, and the institutional structures that contain them are part of the broader fabric of culture, having emerged from culturally inflected attempts to survive disease and avoid death and from responses to illness. Mechanisms have developed which not only provide the framework for delivering medical services but which also shape and define those conditions to be relegated to the medical care system. Descriptions and analyses of the process of the emergence and development of medical systems and the reasons for this within the variety of world cultures define the field known as medical anthropology.[3] As with the development of any institutional system in society, the emergence of medical systems has been accompanied by a range of important secondary developments that shape an anthropology of healing: the determination of what constitutes disease and how that is integrated into the culture and perceived by the patient, the identification of the healer and how he or she functions in a culture, and, finally, how the process of healing occurs within a culture.

## Disease as a Cultural Phenomenon

The concept of disease is multifactoral. Most frequently presented in the medical literature as "an interruption or perversion of function of any of the organs" or "an abnormal state of the body as a whole, continuing for a longer or shorter period," this definition of disease, which is widely accepted, is solely biological in its characterization.[4] Though it does recognize the essential statistical basis for the identification of disease (i.e., that it is a deviation from how the majority of organs or bodies function and therefore does not represent an absolute notion), nonetheless this and similar medical definitions rely purely on statistical deviations of a biophysiological nature as the basic determinant of what constitutes disease.

But in addition to malfunction in physiology, disease is *always* a function of where people live, their social relations, their values, and their technology. This "function" was not unknown to Virchow, who appeared to be convinced that when "medicine" became aware of all it entails, it would become "an anthropology." Virchow's definition of disease is broader in scope and would require that physicians not limit their inquiry of suffering patients to the internal workings of their organs or the external manifestations of dysfunction, but rather that they unravel the human networks of interaction in which they and the patients play their respective roles. While interviewing and examining patients, physicians are privileged in their access to more than just the physical information about the patient; they see intimate aspects of the patient's psychosocial life and his or her social and environmental "ecology."

The significance of this broad access to information about a patient is most readily understood through consideration of the distinction between symptom and sign in the disease process. This distinction is analogous to that between illness and disease. Illness, as with symptom, refers to what the patient experiences. Disease, including its physical manifestation, is never directly experienced as such by the patient. Illness, in contrast, emerges from cultural expectations; that is, it is constructed of beliefs and knowledge which may be situation precise and limited to a particular space and time in social history. For example, hyperactivity did not exist as a disease entity fifty years ago. The fact that it was not classified as disease at that time does not mean that it did not exist. It is probable that hyperactivity was indeed as manifest (by sign) as that which we now consider a disease process, but it simply went unrecognized. Or, perhaps alternatively, new environmental influences, most particularly food coloring and other additives, have created this condition, which to the suffering patient is now seen as an illness. If in fact hyperactivity always existed as a disease in accordance with traditional definitions, then it is interesting to note that the illness component of this was only recently invented.

We have another, more dramatic example in the disease entity of sickle cell anemia. In parts of Africa where this condition prevails, it has not until recently been perceived as an abnormal state. In large part this is because those suffering from it never recognized it as an illness but, even more importantly and contrastively, patients with sickle cell trait were often in an advantageous physiological position to those who did not suffer from the condition. The trait, unlike the full condition which is accompanied by florid symptoms, acts as a prophylaxis against malaria. Hence, to the extent that illness exists as the perception of those suffering from the condition, what must be experienced is a sense of contrast with the majority who do not have the condition, thereby rendering the illness state relative. Consequently, in both the case of illness and symptom (single manifestation of the broader concept of illness) the designation is subjective; it is the state reported by the patient and usually emerges after negotiations with others as to whether or not one is indeed ill and has symptoms to report. In contrast, disease or sign refers to something that is objectively described by the physician. As in a shifting Venn diagram model, there is almost always an overlap to some degree in the diagnosis of disease and illness.

Mental illness is especially characteristic in this regard. As with the physical diseases, some types of mental illness encompass both components of disease and illness quite markedly. The disease component of mental illness can be instanced in a physiological aberration; for example, the existence of a temporal lobe tumor which is clearly evidence of an abnormal physiological process and is experienced by the patient as an illness. But many mental illnesses are not so easily subject to the distinction between disease and illness. These conditions are referred to as functional illnesses and add a complicated wrinkle to the physiological and cultural dimensions of disease. Conditions such as schizophrenia not only do not provide a clear-cut physiological abnormality as a means of comprehending the medical dimensions of the condition but also may not include a subjective or patient-oriented dimension which would be reported by the patient as symptom. Paranoid schizophrenics, for example, may not recognize their own cognitive constructs (regarding adverse forces in the environment that are colluding to destroy them) as symptomatic of an underlying disease process. To these patients this construct is reality and hence their "normal" state is not shared by the majority who manage to avoid turning fantasy in any one instance into reality.

Psychiatrists in their management of functional illnesses rely almost totally on definitions derived from cultural values. Unlike internists, who may resort to laboratory tests to substantiate the existence of a disease process that is compatible with a range of symptoms, psychiatrists are forced to rely on cultural interpretations in their determination of disorders of mood, thought, and behavior. Out of the background of social interactions and general patterns of behavior we must abstract those deviations that are so far removed from the realm of acceptable behavior that they may appropriately be designated as psychiatric disturbances. Psychiatrists are forced to understand, appreciate, and share patient perceptions regarding complicated notions of cause and effect in order to determine the degree of deviation in thinking process and behavior. This requires that psychiatrists not only be sensitive and acutely aware of the cultural panorama of the patient's world but that they become aware also of their own values and opportunities for distortion. Only through this phenomenological method can an "objective" determination be made of the patient's range of behavioral reactions to external stimuli and internal forces. Psychiatrists should understand the logics, linguistics, and symbolic systems of those cultures in which they work.

In addition to the components that illness adds to the disease state and those dimensions created by the functional mental illnesses with regard to deviations in mood, thought, and behavior, the culture often embellishes, dramatizes, or denigrates both physical and mental disease states. An illustration of this is provided by the cultural status of tuberculosis in the 1830s in Europe. This disease, which claimed 17.6 percent of all deaths in 1839, had acquired a status by which ideal beauty was defined.[5] Poetry and drama emerged, preferably and with some expectation, from tuberculosis victims. This in fact was often the case, as with Keats and Chopin, for example, or in the case of the "less creative sex" through the heroines of operas and dramas. In *The Magic Mountain,* Thomas Mann continues this metaphorical association with the characters of Settembrini and Castorp, both of whom experienced a heightening of their inner spiritual selves along with the deterioration of their bodies by the disease.[6] In fact, the more intellectual and gifted were said to be easy prey for tuberculosis; it was associated with spiri-

tualization, euphoria, sensibility, and, for good measure, heightened
sexuality. It was fashionable, for example, for women to drink lemon
juice to inhibit appetite so that they might simulate the appearance of
TB victims.[7] Such women, both the sick and those who could achieve
the pale reflection of such beauty, became models for painters. Though
their skin was pale, their cheeks were flushed and their eyes were said to
"sparkle like diamonds."

Disease metaphors are not always a source for euphoric aesthetic
structuring of social behavior. In *Illness as Metaphor,* Susan Sontag
contrasts the differing perceptions of tuberculosis and cancer in our culture.[8] With cancer, the metaphor is pejorative, as this is a disease condition associated with wasting away, lack of energy, and spiritual and
physical deterioration. Cancer, as Sontag points out, is a disease of
space; it spreads, proliferates, and transmogrifies the physical structure
of the body and, in similar ways, the emotional and spiritual uniqueness
of the individual. Other diseases in western civilization, such as syphilis
and more recently the Acquired Immune Deficiency Syndrome (AIDS),
share this undesirable metaphor. Similarly, in "primitive" cultures certain diseases are also perceived metaphorically as evil. Among the Fore
of New Guinea, *kuru,* a degenerative disease of the central nervous system that is invariably terminated by death after much debilitation and
suffering, provides a focus of social relations around a matrix of sorcery. The victim is considered bewitched and the sequelae to such a diagnosis engender anger, bitterness, recrimination, and revenge, consuming much personal and social energy and resources.[9]

Culture is composed of systems of meaning, including symbols and
myths, by which varied groups of human beings organize their lives,
and medicine, in its practice, encompasses both the cultural and the biological dimensions of humanity. Unfortunately, in the past the literature
stressed two fields of inquiry, the study of culture or the study of medicine, so that anthropology and medicine have been kept apart. Each in
the past has emphasized its own concerns with the human condition.
Similarly, the literature in each of the fields is written to appeal to only
one group or the other. Rarely even now is there an attempt to bridge
the gap between the biological and cultural dimensions which must be
understood more as unifying themes in the determination of the human
condition. But patients are simultaneously both biological and cultural
organisms. For the physician this is particularly important to understand
in order to optimize the health of an individual patient or, for that matter,
to understand epidemiology at any level.

An excellent example of the risks that can occur from misdiagnosis
resulting from lack of sensitivity for the human condition can be made
conspicuous in the examination of the literature concerned with the Chi-

nese cultural context and the Chinese experience with psychosomatic illnesses. The incidence of mental illness in China has always been considered small, fitting into our western notions that the Chinese are a calm and perhaps even a phlegmatic people. But recent studies by both Chinese and western psychiatrists indicate that the Chinese are inclined to somatize psychological problems and express them through physiological disorders.[10] A study of classic Chinese novels leads us to understand that the Chinese have always believed that anger, grief, sorrow, and regret will likely lead people to become ill and die. Ideal women in these novels were not healthy, but smart, beautiful, weak, and easily prone to anxiety and anger, which brought about a yin/yang imbalance in the five elements of gold, wood, water, fire, and earth in their bodies.[11] The traditional strong association between affect and physiological disorders as well as the need to repress emotion and the supreme value of self-control is imparted through training in early childhood. The stigma attached to mental illness by the Chinese has easily led to denial of mental illness by both the patient and his or her family. The psychological mechanism for handling emotional and mental distress therefore becomes that of displacement. One somatizes complaints, allowing "mental illness" to be managed effectively through management of physiological symptoms through traditional medical treatment.

There are further benefits for the doctor and the patient in the somatization of mental illness. As the doctor accepts the sick role as presented by the patient, both healer and the "sick" have an acceptable excuse for the demonstration of affection. Also, it provides the patient with a legitimate excuse to avoid social obligations. Lastly, it creates a mechanism whereby the patient can express indignation about interpersonal relationship or other aspects of his or her life. The most extreme example of this would be suicide but other manifestations such as severe gastrointestinal disturbance would suffice under certain conditions. From the perspective of physicians the advantages are that they need not concern themselves with "placing blame" on other family members, which may be the case were they to diagnose the patient's condition as a mental disorder and thereby seek an appropriate cure. Instead, physicians are in voluntary collusion in the acceptance of the somaticized response as an authentic disease process and avert any allusion of disturbances of the mind or the family as a social system. Nevertheless, despite the advantages in terms of conforming with the strictures of what is acceptable in Chinese society, such cultural limitations severely limit, if not distort, the proper classification and treatment of disease. Because of the sanctions and strictures that a culture imposes on what is acceptable behavior, it narrows considerably the scope of those conditions that can be viewed as diseases. As a result, perception by the patient of his or her condition is ignored unless it can be relegated to a physical sign that is recognized as a disease. Therefore, the distorting effect created by the cultural restrictions can mean that some individuals suffering from illness without the opportunity for somaticization will be forced to either accept the ostracism associated with mental illness or personally absorb suffering the perception of illness and deny the existence of any disease process.

## The Healer in the Context of Culture

To examine the role of the healer as separate from the manner in which a culture conceptualizes disease and illness is artificial and inadequate. Inevitably the latter (that is, those conceptualizations of those conditions which are evidence of the sick state) affect the nature of healing. The role of the healer is very different in a society that maintains a strong mystical or spiritual center to its existence and thereby infuses all of its social forms with a spectrum of religious significances. For instance, in such a culture, epilepsy might be appropriately seen as a disease that relates to a spiritual condition, a closeness to something mystical, prophetic, and transcendental. In contrast, in a western allopathic medical system which places a primacy on scientism, epilepsy is seen as merely a biophysiological process which is subject to predictable laws of science. In either one of these illustrations the role of the healer would not be comparable to the other. In the religiously oriented social system, whether healing is a desirable intervention or not is debatable in the case of the epileptic, for he or she is perceived as close to a transcendental spirit. In such cases the healer is a kind of priest who understands and is in communion with the spirits inhabiting the person in seizure. The contemporary western European, however, sees healers as scientists rigorously trained in neurophysiology and dressed in very formal, if not white, garb. Their apparel emphasizes the "clinical" nature of the intervention and divests them of any claims to spiritual superiority or to any but the most circumstantial linkage to a religious center. It also says that this encounter will be aseptic and impersonal. Obviously these are extreme examples along the spectrum of the ways in which disease may be classified and healers characterized, but they do serve to illustrate most clearly the importance of thinking or connecting the role of the healer with the ways in which origins of illnesses are perceived by the people within a culture.

Western allopathic physicians, whether they are dealing with patients in cultures other than our own or with patients within the variety of subcultures of which our nation is composed, need to understand that the role of the healer is validated in fashions very diverse from their own

training and certification. Among many Native American groups, traditional healing complexes are as valid today as they were in the past, at
least when resorted to in a series of attempts at cure, as we shall see
shortly. To use the example of the Digueño Indians of Southern California, the shaman, or healer, is "chosen" by validation through a series of
personal experiences and he becomes a repository of knowledge and a
master of methods for the control of supernatural forces that affect many
human affairs, most particularly disease and illness. As the shaman is
principally concerned with the supernatural and with healing, his medical education is seen as a mysterious process in which power is derived
from the realm of the supernatural and, therefore, the shaman acts as a
mediator through whom these powers can be used in a variety of ways
for defeating illness.[12] In the selection of the shaman, some emphasis
was placed on the fact that he knew about herbs and other practical
cures, but the primary interest of the community in its selection was the
fact that he exhibited interest in magic and healing and that he was a
gifted dreamer, mainly for prophetic dreams. After prolonged fasting
and a drink of *Datura meteloides,* his hallucinatory dream usually revealed mythic beings and mythic animals. His training and internship
involved working with other shamans, where he learned the art of diagnosing severe illness, always brought on by supernatural powers, and
the interpretation of dreams. Simpler healers such as herb women at-
tended to accidents, sore throats, bruises, inflammations, ear aches, and
so on. Although the Digueño do frequent modern clinics and occasionally consult western physicians, dreams are still regarded as a certain
means of diagnosing illness and persons will become ill due to the
shrinking of traditional responsibilities for performing the proper funeral rites.

It is interesting to note that the Digueño were a particularly pragmatic
people. As with other Native American groups, the powers of the shaman
did not go unexamined by the people of the community. It was essential
that he demonstrate that he could heal, that he was capable of using
supernatural powers in the effective treatment of illness. If in fact he
was unable to accomplish this with a certain degree of success, it would
be considered evidence of the fact that he had always lacked this power.
In the case of the elderly amongst the shamans it was believed that the
power had finally waned as part of the process of growing older. The
fate of the shaman who no longer had this power could be particularly
unfortunate. Not only would he be considered responsible for not being
able to heal a person suffering from an endemic disease, but he might
also be accused of deception; that is, presenting himself as being capable of performing the functions of a shaman when in fact he knew he
had lost that power. Interestingly enough, in those situations where he

was unsuccessful in healing a patient, the shaman would have to provide some explanation for his lack of success, and frequently this would involve ascribing the illness to powers exerted by someone in a foreign territory with perhaps superior supernatural powers. Despite the increasing use of western allopathic medicine, the shaman remains an important force for healing among these people particularly because he is in the best position to integrate mind, body, and spirit for them. The beliefs of the people regarding the etiology of illness also remain rooted in supernatural belief. It is now said among the Digueño that current health problems have been caused by "scientists disturbing the balance of the stars and the earth." [13]

A process that the investigator called "the hierarchy of resort in curative practices" was analyzed in detail from a large body of case histories in the Admiralty Islands of New Guinea in the mid 1960s. [14] The primitive groups known as the Manus wanted to join the western European world, but the area of greatest resistance was that of medical practice because of the emphasis on the connectivity of self to others, to the lineage, to the clan, to totemic animals and plants—all connections crucial to diagnosis and healing and, finally, cure. The role of reversible illness was a moral lesson. In the illness was the punishment; in diagnosis, the judgment; in the cure, rectification and reward. The more acculturated the individual (that is, the more exposure he or she had had to western ways through work or schooling), the more likely he or she would be to go to the western medical clinic first to receive treatment. But this did not preclude the use of traditional healers if in fact the cure expected did not materialize quickly enough. Unacculturated individuals might also avail themselves of western medicine, but *only* after traditional cures failed, for it was acknowledged that there were illnesses of the white people that native medicine might not cure. And, of course, there were indigenous diseases that the white people's medicine could not cure. For example, certain indigenous diseases were seen as the result of travel, which was known to be dangerous because it exposed one to sorcery and illness.

In another study of traditional medicine versus western medicine among the Ningerum of Papua, New Guinea, Robert Welsh discovered that treatment selection through a hierarchy of resort (as shown earlier by Romanucci-Ross) also applied among this indigenous population. [15] Welsh suggests that between the two areas there were differences indicating that in the group he studied, treatment choices and medicinal choices were eclectic and did not appear to reflect a concern with the cultural provenience of the cure. It would seem that cultures also shape the paradigms to be followed in hierarchies of resort in curative practices.

Medical treatments are subject to inflections derived from the paradigms of deeper structures of thought about the universe and the place of humans and objects within it. Our primitive contemporaries' world view suggests that the color and size of medications are related to strength, in compliance with their cultural beliefs regarding these qualities and their association with power. Similarly, personal movement or rest in the illness state is dictated by the best stance for wrestling with the evil of illness caused by infractions of the social code that result in particular manifestations of organic disorders. Although these patients would grant western medicine its superiority in measurement (of temperature or of blood pressure), we fail them since we cannot tell them *why* a particular person got sick while others did not.

## Cultural Differences and Treatment Strategies

Eastern thought, and almost all nonwestern thought, is often characterized as relational, intuitive, synthetic, and passive while negating the finite. In contrast, we postulate that western thought is classificatory, logical, analytical, active, and emphatic and exquisitely descriptive about the finite. Such dichotomies do not serve us very well when we try to explain how and why Easterners handle technology very well and can be quite proficient in "our" science. The extraordinary achievements of the Japanese in contemporary times, particularly in the highly developed technologies of computer and automated systems, would strongly imply that descriptions of thinking processes are highly relativistic and at best a residue of historical curiosity rather than statements about structural differences in the nature of thinking in western as opposed to nonwestern cultures. On the other hand, this analysis of the differences in thinking is perhaps more useful in terms of health, illness, and curing, probably because this is an area of greatest resistance in the acculturation process of primitive societies and in the influence of western ideas on less sophisticated cultures. The western mode of thought translates into the values and the ideology of western medicine, an ideology which emphasizes the value of human mastery over nature, of quantitative measurements, of biomedical causation as temporal and metonymic, and of illness as natural and healing as cultural.

An examination of Japanese values reveals a cultivated intuitive mode with a "this-worldliness" attitude to sensible concrete events; we can see these as depicted by Ukiyo-e artists and find them in delicacies of the changing seasons as seen in Japanese cooking, flower arrangements, and haiku verse. For the Japanese, social relations loom in importance over the person; families and institutions are deeply cherished. The aim of Zen practice is for a realizable worldly goal; that is, for a warrior it was an ever-increasing devotion to a lord, while in today's world it may be to perfect a skill or a style of conduct.

The way these values are transformed into healing practices can be seen most readily in Japanese psychotherapy. One important method of such therapy is referred to as Morita therapy, which is known as "looking inside" for the discovery of guilt and gratitude.[16] This is accomplished by a regimen of prescribed bed rest. The patient is deprived of television, radio, books, and other stimuli for seven days, from 9:00 A.M. until 5:30 P.M.; he or she has to think of the care and kindnesses received and what he or she has done or not done in repayment. The patient must think of interdependence and the trouble that he or she has caused in the fulfillment of an interrelationship. Patients must maximize the other and minimize the self. For Morita therapy the goal is to "see things undistorted, in their original state." Society is an illusion and a critical goal of the therapy is to empty one's self and recognize this illusion.

Interesting observations can be made about the Japanese version of psychotherapy and that used in our own western culture. In many ways it might be argued that the goals of the two are somewhat similar. In Japanese psychotherapy interdependence is valued, and, similarly, it could be argued that a major goal of western psychotherapy is adaptation to society, which would include acceptance by society or the ability to "fit in." Both of these systems of therapy, therefore, would seem to emphasize the cohesiveness and survival of the society with the individual recognizing his or her role within it. But there are important differences. Western psychotherapy presents itself as having an objective of self-actualization; that is, the development of the individual means the recognition of his or her uniqueness. In contrast, the Japanese approach always requires the submission to a higher order, that is, maximization of the other and interdependence. In fact, on closer examination of western psychotherapy, even self-actualization may be nothing more than a facade that is easily crumbled when it comes into conflict with the social process. The underlying currents in western psychotherapy are strongly directed toward conformity. The difference rests in the fact that for the ideals of Morita therapy the patient must recognize that society is an illusion, still emphasizing interdependence and the other. In western psychotherapy the patient must tap in on some notions of self-actualization but finally join the illusion of society so that we can all make it reality.[17]

Religion and other belief systems affect how one thinks about healing, and this is another focus of significant difference between East and West. In the East, religion and healing have been very closely linked. Buddha was healed when he saw a sick man; hence, becoming a Buddhist is seen as a healing process of body and mind until one is saved. Suffering is a derivative of craving and desire. One must get rid of lust (an excess of wind), anger (an excess of bile), and delusion (an excess of phlegm). Illness can teach you and lead you to your liberation. As a result the healing process is a metaphor for spiritual growth. This is in contra-distinction to the methods that would be available for getting rid of bodily diseases. Such methods would and do include the use of herbs, specific foods, and surgery if need be. Hospitals are also for the practice of compassion. In the West, Christ was a healer as much as he was a moralist; in the New Testament there are many illustrations of Christ di-rectly healing the blind and the infirm. In modern times Christian Sci-ence emphasizes the primacy of thought as the cause of all evil and ills; thoughts along with confessions and community prayer constitute the process of healing and cure.[18]

However, as in other areas, a little knowledge about the role of culture in illness and healing can be misleading. Many a scientist who has be-come a convert to understanding the etiologies of disease and illness that are probably cultural tends to err toward cultural explanations when physiological research might be more to the point both for learning about a disease and developing effective methods of treatment. This ten-dency to accept cultural etiologies is most pronounced in the area of ab-errations of behavior. For example, some scientists who have witnessed a case of arctic hysteria (piblokto) have described it immediately and unequivocably as a cultural disorder. Piblokto provides the diagnostician with signs of deep depression, glossalalia, and hysterical behavior that readily transform into hostile, threatening, and violent acts with delu-sions of cannibalism. Piblokto, when investigated with the calcium hy-pothesis as a possible explanation, becomes quite a different entity, both biological *and* cultural, with interesting transformations.[19] It would appear that the cold, uniform darkness of the Eskimo habitat results in understimulation of all the senses, which is an important component in understanding the disease process. The other component is calcium defi-ciency due to the lack of Vitamin D and ultraviolet rays. Where these are lacking, plasma calcium decreases. Below a certain threshold, stand-ing potentials at neural synapses tend to break down, releasing minute amounts of transmitter substances causing spasms that are not cortically controlled.

In an interesting transformation from biological to cultural, the dra-matic behavior of the "patient" is mimicked by the shaman. He achieves a physiological state exhibiting similar behavioral symptoms by self-induced understimulation, lack of food and liquids, self-induced suffer-ing through beating administered by self and others, and finally hyperventilation. This helps him to achieve an "altered state" so that he can become an effective healer. It is a state mimicked also by the lay public (nonshamans) for the management of personal stress. Piblokto then can be explained either as neural physiology, mimetic behavior in shamanic ritual, or coping behavior. Therefore, cultural dimensions as manifested in the mimesis provide only one explanation for the development of this condition. In fact, it would appear that piblokto in the truly affected individual is the result of various deprivations affecting the neurophysiological system of the patient.

Another example of biological and cultural illness is that of the *tarantismo* cult in southern Italy. This phenomenon was studied in great detail and analyzed in depth by an anthropologist and a team of physicians, psychiatrists, and ethnologists.[20] Although the real bite of the tarantula can have definable physiological consequences, there are in fact a large number of *tarantati,* of afflicted persons, who have not been bitten by a tarantula. The symptoms as manifested in the behavior of those who are putatively afflicted are similar to those who have actually been bitten. The ritual cure involves music, with a particular emphasis on the use of percussion instruments, the display of brightly colored clothes, food, the company of others to aid in the healing, and dancing by the *tarantato,* often to the point of physical exhaustion. The age, sex, and social status of the afflicted give the participant audience the clue as to what sort of tarantula caused the "illness." For example, the classification includes tarantulas of envy, of lust, or of greed. It can readily be surmised that this illness and ritual cure can be directed to a physiological affliction or a person stressed beyond endurance in a highly rigid culture. The cure, which includes food and entertainment for all present, is an exercise in social and personal reintegration in an aesthetic context.

In this case as well as the earlier one involving piblokto the scientist who adheres strongly to the cultural explanation for the illness will ignore a very real biochemical basis in those individuals who are actually bitten. By the same token the biophysiological explanation is not complete. It is likely an explanation that is only applicable to a small percentage of those actually presenting themselves as *tarantati.* In many ways, both of these examples piblokto and *tarantismo*—suggest that illness in a society can be viewed in much the same way in which we examine social texts. That is, an illness is clearly more than a biophysiological condition and more than a cultural reaction to specific happenings. The combination of both is a statement of the way in which a culture has institutionalized certain behaviors, symptom complexes, and diseases to essentially tell a story, a story of what events have certain kinds of significances and thereby justify certain responses. Individual diseases that are mixed with a major cultural overlay essentially tell a story about the culture in much the same way that a myth or a dance serves to communicate cognitive as well as affective qualities that are basic and valued in the culture, thereby allowing expressivity in the actions and behaviors of indigenous people. When seen from this perspective the western scientist who has nearly effectively divested disease of its story-telling or communicative role misses the point by reducing a condition such as piblokto to either a biophysiological explanation or a purely cultural phenomenon. It is the integration of both in varying degrees that finally provides a full understanding of illnesses and the role of healers in various cultures.

## The Impact of Cultural Understanding on Western Medicine

What can we learn from folk medical practice that will aid our understanding of health care delivery in complex societies? Any culture permits illness to play various roles, such as asserting individual needs and eliciting certain kinds of behavior from others, as we have indicated above. Illness is therefore a negotiable event. So there are illnesses that can be ignored or those that can be exaggerated. Persons who consider themselves ill will consult others and, finding a reasonable consensus, begin a "journey cure." How personal notions of systems balance are operant in the maintenance of health relate as much to what is observed in primitive and peasant cultures as in complex cultural settings. People who do not use words such as "homeostasis" have, nevertheless, a very good sense of it.[21]

There are two major reasons why it is important for western physicians to understand more about the range of different diseases and illnesses that exist in various cultural contexts and the ways in which a culture has institutionalized systems for dealing with these conditions either in a healing manner or as a mechanism for social reintegration. First, a knowledge of other cultures will enable western medicine to become an important method of treatment for those suffering throughout the world and, second, such knowledge would sensitize western physicians to ways in which they affect the discontinuance of certain treatments that are ineffective or harmful to the patient. With regard to the first of these, western physicians will not achieve any degree of success in their desire to impart a respect for our notions of health and preventive medicine and cure to other societies if they ignore the cultural context and all the implications for social relations involved in notions of health and illness. Furthermore, in some ways of greater importance, to learn the world view of the culture or subculture means that the physician will understand the patient, because the locus of culture is *in the person*. Therefore, a good model for the introduction of cultural change, especially if one seeks the best of both worlds, is a typical doctor in a Chinese province.[22] Typically, Chinese doctors are elected for medical training by villagers who trust their character and intelligence. After three months' training these doctors will have introduced vaccines for small pox, measles, and polio (since 1970 there has been a 92 to 100 percent drop in these diseases) as well as vitamins, antibiotics, and traditional Chinese medicine such as acupuncture and moxibustion (heat for acupuncture points whereby the stimulation is supplied by a slow-burning plant, *Artemisia vulgaris*). They will have learned the pharmacopoeia of herbs, roots, minerals, and animal substances, knowledge usually imparted by a learned old woman. They are assisted by experts from time to time who may adjust an IUD, treat fractures and burns, and do some dental work. They take correspondence courses from an institute to augment their training. Since in their person and practice they embody therapies of East and West that work and since they are trusted as individuals and healers, anything they introduce is acceptable to their patients. The individual who volunteers to be a cultural mediator in medical care may not be the most liked or trusted person of the group; patients may therefore be unable to establish the rapport necessary to begin a reformation of medical practices. In some parts of the world, such as Italian rural areas, physicians include folk healers in the referral system.

A plurality of medical systems is one of the universals of medical care. So, too, are notions of balance (yin and yang, or hot and cold as in South America), notions of public health (which may have little in common with our western notions of public health), and notions of purity and pollution. A knowledge of other cultures, their plurality of medical systems, and the ideologies and values that sustain them can be of great value in efforts to help other societies benefit from the great strides we have made in western medicine. These other systems, too, have aspects that are effective and can be empirically verified—a pharmacology, for example.[23]

Is there anything we can learn from nonwestern systems to increase our own medical effectiveness? An interesting area of overlap is the placebo effect, an element present in every medical system. In fact, it has been suggested that as much as 35 to 60 percent of the effectiveness of contemporary biomedicine may be attributable to the placebo effect. In the treatment of angina pectoris alone it has been suggested that 70 to 90 percent effectiveness has been reported by enthusiastic placebo pushers.[24] The placebo effect includes not only the therapeutic deception of a pharmacologically or biomedically inert substance that affects the outcome of disease or illness, but ritual as well. This may include more than just the actions of the shaman but also the very intricate ritual associated with modern surgery and the use of the operating room.

The second benefit for western physicians that can be achieved by understanding other cultures is sensitivity for the limitations of our own treatments in the care of patients. It is easy to look into the past with a critical eye at the tortures that have been perpetrated on the sick for centuries. Methods such as the use of bleeding, purging, and excrements from various animals, the whipping of the insane to relieve them of possessed devils, and removal of the colon with no pathology are only a few of the examples of bizarre medical practices that existed in our own culture not too many years ago. Similarly, it would be easy to look at the explanations provided in various cultures for illnesses and the ways in which those cultures handled them and take a superior stance regarding contemporary developments. But the lesson that is to be learned is not so much the fact that bizarre medical practices exist and cultures have unusual ways of understanding illness (in some cases either partially or wholly correct) but that in our own understanding of illness and methods for treatment we are also limited. We are influenced by ideologies, myths, and the symbolic significance of certain kinds of interventions (for example, surgery in many cases) which the future will surely unravel and examine with an equally critical eye. The lesson that seems to be most important is twofold, first, the concepts of disease, illness, and the roles of the healer are complex, as exemplified in various cultures; second, a heightened sensitivity is created to those methods of treatment that are used in an unquestioned fashion essentially for the care of patients that may be equally to their detriment, as some of the medically bizarre practices in the past.

## Conclusion

Medicalization, a term we hear with some frequency, can be described in a basic way as the structuring of information by the providers of health care. But the process derives even greater force and more lasting effects from medical advertising and the profession's throw-away journals from which the practitioner (as well as the rest of us) gets much current information. The advertising world is a repository of all techniques of persuasion as the consumer is assailed with juxtapositions of medications and of dietary supplements with powerful symbols of attractiveness, sexuality, and affluence. And the culture itself structures and processes information, but it also contains all the historical residues that in time accumulate and influence structuring and processing. Within our problem orientation, medicalization can be viewed, and is viewed by many, as an attempt by power holders to leave the dependent patient little acceptable choice. Perhaps our western allopathic medicine will, as it has in the past, assimilate what is scientifically valid into its own body of knowledge while broadening its hypotheses about health and behavior in the cultural context. We share with cultural groups of less complexity and less internal diversity shifting game strategies in confronting illness to regain health.[25]

We referred to the Manus' illness, intervention, and cure "task" as basically sociomoral, and we have noted that it is believed to achieve results. So, too, with the appropriation of the arctic hysteria syndrome by the shaman for purposes of healing which, like all other healing ventures, works much if not all of the time and with some if not all afflicted persons who seek the shamanic cure. The same observations could be made for the ritual cure of those "bitten" by the tarantula. In these three exemplary cases there is meaning in illness and cure in terms of problem identification and analysis, the support of the social network, and the task of the performance. Lévi-Strauss makes the case that the shaman, along with the methodology shared by him and the patient, alters physiological processes through control of mental processes, dissolving the boundary between self and other and offering the patient a path for reintegration into the group.[26] He compares the shaman to the psychoanalyst who allows the conscious and unconscious to merge. This is accomplished through a shared symbolic system, and because of the performance, the patient calls into play the group's sentiments and symbolic representations to embody them in real experience. The key to this social process is the relationship between symbolism and the consequential healing.

In this era of ever-escalating medical malpractice cases, which are reputed to reflect the breakdown in the physician-patient relationship, there is clearly a need for contemporary physicians to understand the importance of the relationship between symbol and healing. The past fifty years have witnessed major advances in technological developments for the understanding of medical diseases and practice, but with these advances there seems to have been a nearly commensurate regression in the contemporary western physician's understanding of the nature of his or her relationship with the patient and how that relationship fits within the broad symbolic system that constitutes society. The understanding of other cultures that rely more heavily on the art of healing can teach us ways to reintroduce this critical feature into the care and treatment of the patient living in a modern cultural context. In the perspective of the contemporary medical scene it is this third benefit that western medicine can derive from understanding the anthropology of medical care that may finally become the most important aspect in the years to come if medicine is to maximize all of the knowledge and forces that it has at its command to enhance the care of patients and continue strongly in the direction of greater understanding of the biophysiological and cultural dimensions of disease and illness in the care of patients.

## Notes

1. See chap. 1, this volume.

2. Carleton Chapman, *Physicians, Law, and Ethics* (New York: New York University Press, 1984).

3. Lola Romanucci-Ross, Daniel Moerman, and Laurence Tancredi, eds., *The Anthropology of Medicine: From Culture to Method* (South Hadley, Mass.: Bergin and Garvey, 1983).

4. Thomas Lathrop Stedman, *Stedman's Medical Dictionary: Illustrated*, 24th ed. (Baltimore: Williams and Wilkins, 1982), 403.

5. G. Melvyn Howe, *Man, Environment and Disease in Britain* (New York: Barnes and Noble, 1972), 179.

6. Thomas Mann, *The Magic Mountain* (New York: Random House, 1927).

7. Rene DuBos and Jean DuBos, *The White Plague: Tuberculosis, Man and Society* (Boston: Little, Brown, 1952).

8. Susan Sontag, *Illness as Metaphor* (New York: Farrar, Strauss and Giroux, 1978).

9. Shirley Lindenbaum, *Kuru Sorcery* (Palo Alto: Mayfield, 1979).

10. Wen-Shing Tseng, "The Nature of Somatic Complaints among Psychiatric Patients: The Chinese Case," *Comprehensive Psychiatry* 16 (1975): 237–245; Arthur Kleinman, "Depression, Somatization and the New Cross-Cultural Psychiatry," *Social Science and Medicine* 11 (1977): 3–10; Jen-Yi Wang, "Psychosomatic Illness in the Chinese Cultural Context," in *The Anthropology of Medicine*, ed. Romanucci-Ross, Moerman, and Tancredi, 298–318.

11. Wang, "Psychosomatic Illness."

12. Spencer L. Rogers and Lorraine Evernham, "Shamanistic Healing among the Digueño Indians of Southern California," in *The Anthropology of Medicine*, ed. Romanucci-Ross, Moerman, and Tancredi, 103–118.

13. Ibid., 116.

14. Lola Romanucci-Ross, "The Hierarchy of Curative Practices: The Admiralty Islands, Melanesia," *Journal of Health and Social Behavior* 10 (1969): 201–209.

15. Robert Welsh, "Traditional Medicine and Western Medical Options among the Ningerum," in *The Anthropology of Medicine*, ed. Romanucci-Ross, Moerman, and Tancredi, 32–53.

16. Takie Lebra, "The Social Mechanism of Guilt and Shame: The Japanese Case," *Anthropological Quarterly* 44, no. 4 (October 1971): 241–255; George DeVos, *Socialization for Achievement: Essay on the Cultural Psychiatry of the Japanese* (Los Angeles: University of California Press, 1973), 478–479.

17. Laurence Tancredi and Andrew Slaby, "Ethical Issues in Mental Health Care," in *Medical Ethics and the Law; Implications for Public Policy*, ed. M. D. Hiller (Cambridge: Ballinger, 1982), 283–302; Andrew Slaby and Laurence Tancredi, *Collusion for Conformity* (New York: Jason Aronson, 1975).

18. Stefan Zweig, *Mental Healers: Franz Anton Mesmer, Mary Baker Eddy, Sigmund Freud* (New York: Frederick Ungar, 1962).

19. Edward F. Foulks, *The Arctic Hysterias of the North Alaskan Eskimo*. Anthropo-

logical Studies, no. 10, ed. David H. Maybury-Lewis (Washington, D.C.: American Anthropological Association, 1976).

20. Ernesto DeMartino, *La terra del rimorso* (Milan: Il Saggiatore, 1961).

21. Lola Romanucci-Ross, "Medicalization and Metaphor," in *The Use and Abuse of Medicine,* ed. M. W. de Vries, R. L. Berg, and M. Lipkin, Jr. (New York: Praeger, 1982), 173–174.

22. Doris Howell, M.D., personal communication.

23. Memory Elvin-Lewis, "The Antibiotic and Healing Potential of Plants Used for Teeth Cleaning," in *The Anthropology of Medicine,* ed. Romanucci-Ross, Moerman, and Tancredi, 201–220; James W. Herrick, "The Symbolic Roots of Three Potent Iroquois Medicinal Plants," in ibid., 134–155; Nina L. Etkin and Paul J. Ross, "Malaria, Medicine and Meals: Plant Use among the Hausa and Its Impact on Disease," in ibid., 231–260.

24. Daniel E. Moerman, "Physiology and Symbols: The Anthropological Implications of the Placebo Effect," in ibid., 156–167.

25. Romanucci-Ross, "Medicalization and Metaphor," 177, 179–180.

26. Claude Lévi-Strauss, *Structural Anthropology* (New York: Doubleday, 1967).

# 10. *The Lost Secret of Ancient Medicine*

**Guido Majno**

Surely the lost secrets of ancient medicine are many; we learn about them only when they are retrieved. Auscultation was retrieved (or rediscovered) by Laennec two thousand years after Hippocrates.[1] Asthmatics would have avoided much suffering for nineteen centuries if their physicians had known a passage of Pliny the Elder extolling the virtues of ephedra "for those short of breath" (ephedrin resurfaced in China in 1924).[2] The uniquely soothing properties of the crocus (*Colchicum*) during acute attacks of gout were forgotten for about fifteen hundred years.[3] What other gems lie buried under piles of millennial rubble?

I do not know about other lost herbs or roots, but I do know about one lost secret, a major one, which had been passed along for thousands of years and then began fading away a few decades ago. It is a truth so simple that I hesitated to mention it, but I chose to write about it anyway because it explains to a large extent the present wave of antimedical feelings. It is, in fact, the basic message of medical history. If I were asked to condense the teachings of a hundred volumes of medical history into three lines, I would write this in flaming letters: *medicine existed thousands of years before it could offer any scientific help to patients, because sick people need, first of all,* ATTENTION: *a great deal of specific, focused, caring attention.* In the days of Hippocrates, physicians had little else to offer except intense attention, and yet they became famous. Modern physicians, of course, still care, but they have little time for the focused attention so critical to the patient. In more scientific terms, the physician is the primal drug, a drug that can be overdosed or underdosed (and even have side effects).[4] Today the dose is dwindling to homeopathic levels.

How and why did this happen? To answer this question we should find out how people coped with disease before there was any scientific medicine. We will do this by visiting the Navajo tribe, where ancestral practices still function, and Dr. Homer Holland, who practiced in Westfield, Massachusetts, around 1840 with the benefit of some anatomy but little else that we could call scientific. And then we will compare these two settings with the medicine that we all know.

## Navajo Medicine

The Navajo met the challenge of physical and spiritual suffering by creating (hundreds and perhaps thousands of years ago) healers who rely primarily on what we would call symbolic cures.[5] Most other tribes have followed a similar path, but the approach to healing among the Navajo is unique: their ceremonial life is almost exclusively devoted to recovering health, and the healing ceremonies themselves are extremely elaborate.

Today a Navajo who is involved in an accident and is physically injured will usually be taken to the nearest hospital; this applies, as far as I have seen, also to medicine men. But a traditional Navajo who feels unwell will first consult a special type of expert known as a diagnostician. Once the disease is diagnosed in Navajo terms, if it is severe enough the proper treatment will be taken over by a medicine man.

Some diagnosticians pronounce their verdict after having gazed into a crystal. Others are known as hand-tremblers; they perform during a self-induced trance. In that condition they violently shake their arm at the patient and the hand finally points to the part that is in trouble. Years ago my wife and I had a nasty car accident just before leaving for the Navajo reservation, so we took this opportunity to get ourselves diagnosed. We were taken to an eighty-year-old hand-trembler, a woman who spoke no English (we had an interpreter). She did inquire about our injuries, but this was clearly not her main interest. There was much chanting and praying with eyes closed, and eventually she let us know the nature of our disease: the sun and the highway had conspired against us. This could be treated with a symbolic offering and a healing ritual that involved taking a potion made with herbs specially gathered for us at sunrise and laced with prayers specific to our particular problem. The potion had to be taken by all those present, including the friends who had driven us there—no exemption admitted. This is a typically Navajo procedure, whereby the attention focused on the patient is instantly multiplied.

Note the basic philosophy of this medicine. Our disease was not represented by our wounds; the wounds were just a consequence, too simple to consider—anybody can treat a wound. For that you can go to the nearest hospital. The real disease was the fact that we had an accident. I am not sure that the sun really conspired, but considering the time of the day, blinding by the sun could have been part of the problem. In any event, the point is that the diagnostician was looking for a deeper cause to the accident. This is good medicine. I am reminded of the same thought expressed by one of my heroes in American medical education, Alan Gregg. In one of his essays he discusses the multiple causes of disease, precisely in relation to a car accident:

> I doubt if I could exaggerate my feelings regarding the stupidity we show in so frequently assuming that one result is due to only one cause. We ought to use the word "why" in the plural and ask "Whys is this patient in a coma?" . . . A particular case of a fractured jaw in a sailor may be the result of convergent causes—no letters from home, too much alcohol, the loan of a car by a friend, a dark night, an oncoming car on a road covered with ice at a curve, the fact that the left-hand rule is used in the British Isles, new brake linings, a skid, and a telephone pole . . . Take out any one of these whys and the accident would not have occurred.[6]

To my wife and me this episode was an adventure of the mind; to a Navajo it would have been an essential part of the healing process— peace for the soul while the wounds healed; time to think about what caused the accident. To the hand-trembler—between preliminary talks, herb gatherings, preparations, the ritual, and the aftermath—it meant the better part of one day.

What if the hand-trembler had concluded that we required a major healing ceremony? That would have become a full-time undertaking, unlikely to be accomplished within the three weeks at our disposal. The first step toward organizing a ceremony is to find the medicine man (or, more precisely, the *Hataatii*, "singer") who knows the appropriate "sing": Beautyway, Flintway, Shootingway, Mountainway, Coyoteway, or any other of the fifty or so still extant on the reservation.[7] The singer might live a hundred miles away. He (singers are almost always male) must be located, then a mutually convenient time must be found, and the fee must be arranged in terms of money, jewelry, livestock, or other belongings. Ceremonies can last from one to nine days, or more correctly nights; the entire family, relatives, and friends are invited to enhance the effect of the ceremony; food must be provided for everybody. Although the patient is helped by contributions of a large supporting group, the total expense can be considerable: thousands of dollars. The singer's fee must be seen in the perspective of his contribution. The entire ceremony must be recited and sung *by heart*. To learn by heart nine whole nights of performance cost the singer about fifteen years of training with an elder, a memory effort that would make our medical students shudder. The performance must be flawless: any slip would destroy its effectiveness. Should memory fail there is nobody there to suggest the next line; worse yet, in the audience there may well be another medicine man who has come to lend moral support, perhaps rehearse his own memory baggage, and incidentally check for flaws. We have seen the method at work: as one medicine man (about sixty years old) recited hour after hour, his older teacher, who happened to be around, sat by him and sang along in perfect unison. This memory effort has few parallels in the world; it is matched only in India of times past when the entire Vedas were learned by heart.[8]

The actual healing ceremony, the sing, is held in a special, conse crated dwelling (hogan): it includes songs, prayers (at times repeated by the patient), myth telling, the administration of symbolic drugs, and above all the now-famous sand paintings.[9] A careful study of these ceremonies, carried out by a California psychiatrist, showed that they are consistently built according to a scheme in five stages: purification, evocation, identification, transformation, and release.[10] Nothing is left to chance. I just wish I could transmit the intensity of emotions in the dimly lit hogan as the singer chants his lines to the accompaniment of a rattle:

> In beauty may I dwell
> In beauty may I walk
> In beauty may my male kindred dwell
> In beauty may my female kindred dwell
> In beauty may it rain on my young men
> In beauty may it rain on my young women
> In beauty may it rain on my chiefs
> In beauty may it rain on us

> In beauty may our corn grow
> On the trail of pollen may it rain
> In beauty before us, may it rain
> In beauty below us, may it rain
> In beauty above us, may it rain
> In beauty all around us, may it rain . . .

Details of these ancient ceremonies can be found in a number of excellent books.[11] We must now concentrate on the essence: does Navajo
medicine work, and if so, why?

It certainly works for the Navajo. The superiority of western medicine
is recognized for healing bodily ills (clinics on the reservation are over-
loaded), but a Navajo lady who has had her gallbladder surgically removed for stones may then elect to have a traditional ceremony sung
over her to restore her life to balance. Non-Navajo physicians on the reservation have long recognized the need for both approaches: we have
seen a modern hospital with a hogan built in its center, where the singers take over after the white coats. The Navajo feel that the treatment by
western medicine is not complete.

What are the missing ingredients, in the eyes of the Navajo? I believe
they can be reduced to two. One is symbolic healing. In our view this
might go under the name of psychotherapy, but we must not forget that
the separation of body and soul is largely a product of our religions: for
the primal mind, life includes body and soul and disease cannot separate
them.[12] Sanity includes the sky, the rain, and everything else that lives
all around, not just family and neighbors, but also the corn, the trees,
and the rocks, which means the psychotherapy works also as bodily
therapy.

The other ingredient is intense focus on the patient: attention again.
Symbolic healing cannot be squeezed into a ten-minute pill. The medicine man can be involved with his patient for the better part of two weeks
on the occasion of a single ceremony, with a total active role on the
order of one hundred hours. His time with the patient is spent in a manner adapted to Navajo culture. We Anglos would expect the healer to ask
us many questions, even very personal ones; to the stoic, self-contained
Navajo this would be inappropriate. If a doctor is obliged to ask many
questions, it means that "he does not know."

This element of time devoted to the treatment is perceived as essential. In 1977, as we visited Phoenix, the newspapers reported that a
group of Navajo workers had gone on strike. Their demands: they wanted
company benefits to include, besides Blue Cross and Blue Shield, the
medicine man and his ceremonies. Questioned by journalists they re-
plied: "The singer spends several days with us; he finds out what is

wrong. The Anglo doctors spend three minutes with us and give us a pill. What can they learn about us in three minutes?"

It may seem, at first sight, that Navajo medicine belongs to fairy tales. Our medicine has no use for crystal gazers or hand-tremblers. But there is a bigger picture. The Navajo recognized, in their own Indian way, the human need for ceremony, the reassuring function of ritual. We practice ritual too, under selected circumstances of life: marriage, birth, graduation, Sunday church. Healing is left out, although we have, as human beings, quite the same basic needs as the Navajo. The Navajo can feel healed by penicillin if they are also ritually restored to the world around them. Our world is rather different; but when we are sick, who helps us make peace with it?

Above all, the Navajo discovered that a sick person can be helped by becoming the focus of attention, and they provide it in the manner that is appropriate for their culture.

## Ancient Medicine, Western Style

By the mid 1800s, with a tradition of at least twenty-two hundred years, western medicine was scarcely more advanced and probably much more harmful than Navajo medicine. Even surgery was a near-catastrophic procedure before anesthesia (1846) and antisepsis (1867). The only effective drugs available at large were opium and occasional leaves of the foxglove for those who knew how to use them. If any significant therapy was accomplished its benefits were wiped out by bleeding, purging, vomiting, and the sinister habit of starving as a cure.[13] The lot of the patient had not really improved since Hippocrates; in some respects it was worse, because horrible new poisons such as mercury had been introduced. Judging from its clinical accomplishments, the medical profession should have died away.

The very fact that medicine did not die away suggests that some other factor must have balanced its negative impact. The factor obviously is care and all that the term implies. See how a practitioner in Massachusetts spent his time in 1840, judging from the entries in his ledger for October of that year:[14]

> October 6—Francis Matson. Attended all night        no pay
> October 8—Edwin B., to splinting limb and attend all night
>            $6.00
> October 8—Mr. White. To visit and attend all night previous
>        he died        $1.75
> October 10—To attend all day and night        $6.00
> October 11—For sundry visits and attend all day and night    $5.00

This means that Dr. Holland spent four out of those five nights at the home of a patient. He even stayed through the death of one, a gesture that the family was not likely to forget. Today the notion of going to a patient's funeral is worthy of publication.[15]

The citizens of Westfield did not realize it, but the help offered by Dr. Holland had very little to do with his training. Most of the time he was helpful despite his knowledge. His drug was human care.

And so the profession survived.

## Medicine Today

When scientific medicine began to perform its healing miracles (only forty or fifty years ago) there was a marvelous opportunity. Ancient medicine had discovered the secret of helping souls. Now it was possible to help bodies as well, thanks to tons of knowledge, chemicals, and machines.

It did not quite work out that way. The new generation of healers was carried away by the physical problems, in fact by anything that could be measured. Spiritual concerns are hard to measure.[16] It was assumed that if the body is healed the rest would somehow follow.

Before long the public began to realize that something was missing. We are now in the midst of a rising antimedical tide, while scores of supposedly "holistic" would-be do-gooders move in to fill the vacuum.[17] At the latest count there are seventy alternative forms of medicine.[18] They certainly have the secret cure—time—and with it they can offer enough hope and smiles to heal 85 percent of all patients.[19]

If we want to reverse the trend we must find out why twentieth-century physicians went off course. The answer is that they did so under tremendous pressures.

The problems begin in medical school. The old ways are very difficult to teach; nobody yet has found a way to teach the human approach. Altschule has said, with characteristic irony, that "it cannot be taught— although it can be learned."[20] The few lectures on ethics or other "humanities" in the medical curriculum still look like pieces of china in a bull shop. How can one bend nature into a given fold, short of turning medical school into a sort of seminary? To the twentieth-century mind, anyway, these are soft concerns. Science is made of hard facts; the battle between hard and soft is quickly over.

The number of facts to learn is another obsession. In the days of Dr. Holland there was not much to read; nothing really new or helpful was being published. Success was based on human qualities and experience; both, with some luck, improved automatically with time. Today, obsolescence is automatic; physicians are flooded daily with new facts that could be critical. New papers are published at the rate of about two per second; just the list of the yearly papers weighs eighty pounds.[21] If a physician learns, or forgets, the wrong facts or the wrong drugs, trigger-happy patients will drag him or her to court to claim damages in the range of millions.

The environment of hospitals is hardly more conducive to spiritual values. The day is dominated by mechanical worries, dials, buttons, and computers, all of which are essential and even vital, but none gives access to the patient's feelings. There are no standard tests for fear, anguish, or unhappiness. Because time is money, which it undeniably is, the time given to an individual patient must be reduced to the minimum in the name of efficiency. The time is measured in minutes, barely enough to get across the key facts. The pressure of time is drilled into the physician from the very beginning: in some services, residents are required to sleep just enough so that their judgment will be only slightly impaired. This comes to five hours of sleep, but there has been some discussion that four might be enough, as the military believes.[22] A worn-out physician is not the likeliest source of empathy.

Hospital architecture raises its own set of problems. It is difficult to rise above the daily routine when the eye cannot catch a glimpse of the sky. Many offices and even patient rooms have no windows. The importance of an opening to the sky must have been appreciated even in the days of the cavemen; brave new architects, in search of new ideas, abolished windows. Perhaps there is hope now that the point of view of the cavemen can be supported by a measurement: it turns out that patients are better off (*measurably* better off) if they have a window offering a natural view.[23]

Society may have reasons to complain about physicians, but physicians themselves are prisoners of a tough reality. This vicious circle must be broken.

## Is There a Remedy?

The message of history, as I have tried to decipher it, is that scientific therapy has eroded the human care which has always been a key part of the healing process.

Young medical graduates, brought up in the system, may find it difficult or impossible to fight the trend.

Maybe so, but there is hope. Awareness of the problem is a first step toward solving it.

I can also offer a practical suggestion. It may be impossible to stretch minutes into hours, but the quality of those minutes can certainly be improved. For the best way to do so, I propose to turn back one hundred years and meet the model physician of that time, indeed of all times, Sir William Osler.

Osler published his famous textbook *The Principles and Practice of Medicine* in 1892, when therapy was almost nil. Osler could do very, very little to physically help his patients. The impotence of his medicine was so shocking that the countershock still echoes around the world: in 1897 a layman, Frederick T. Gates, happened to read Osler's treatise while on vacation; he was so appalled by the lack of available scientific and therapeutic knowledge that he advised John D. Rockefeller to create the Rockefeller Institute of Medical Research. It was dedicated four years later.[24] No more is needed to portray the medicine practiced by Osler. Most of what he did was wrong or useless. Yet he is remembered as one of the greatest, most caring physicians next to Hippocrates.

He had not yet lost the secret of ancient medicine.

New physicians have at their command a formidable set of effective therapies. Think how high they could fly if they also had the wings of Sir William Osler.

## Notes

1.  For the practice of auscultation in Hippocratic medicine, see G. Majno, *The Healing Hand—Man and Wound in the Ancient World* (Cambridge: Harvard University Press, 1975), 158.

2.  For the saga of ephedra and its rediscovery, see ibid., 349ff. and 527, notes 136, 140.

3.  J. S. Goodwin and J. M. Goodwin, "The Tomato Effect: Rejection of Highly Efficacious Therapies," *Journal of the American Medical Association* 251 (1984): 2387.

4.  The concept of "the physician as drug" is amply discussed in an excellent book by psychiatrist Michel Balint, *The Doctor, His Patient and the Illness* (New York: International University Press, 1973).

5.  The best analysis of Navajo healing practices is offered by a California psychiatrist: D. Sandner, *Navajo Symbols of Healing* (New York: Harcourt Brace Jovanovich, 1979).

6.  A. Gregg, *For Future Doctors* (Chicago: University of Chicago Press, 1957), 81.

7.  The number of fifty surviving sings available on the Navajo reservation is probably optimistic. The medicine men are getting along in years and they are not being replaced. School obligations prevent interested children (the few that might choose that path) from following the elders and memorizing the ceremonies. See D. M. Brugge and C. J. Frisbie, eds., *Navajo Religion and Culture—Selected Views. Papers in Honor of Leland C. Wyman* (Santa Fe: Museum of New Mexico Press, 1982).

8.  For memorization in India, see Majno, *The Healing Hand,* 269, note 1, and 512, note 36.

9.  An excellent treatise on so-called sand paintings has appeared recently: Leland C. Wyman, *Southwest Indian Drypainting* (Albuquerque: University of New Mexico Press, 1983).

10.  See Sandner, *Navajo Symbols,* 83.

11.  For references to Navajo ceremonials, see ibid.; Wyman, *Southwest Indian Drypainting;* and Brugge and Frisbie, *Navajo Religion and Culture.*

12. For body and soul in Indian thought, see J. Highwater, *The Primal Mind: Vision and Reality in Indian America* (New York: Meridian Books, New American Library, 1981), 135, passim.

13. For the use of starvation as a cure, see Majno, *The Healing Hand,* 179, 182, 188, 257, 291, 297, 304, 310, 335, 337, 355, 419.

14. Account Book of Dr. Homer Holland, Physician of Westfield, Mass. (1840–1841). Manuscript located at the Research Library of Old Sturbridge Village, Sturbridge, Mass.

15. P. Irvine, "The Attending at the Funeral," *New England Journal of Medicine* 312 (1985): 1074–1075.

16. There is an "empathy scale," but not much can be expected of it. See R. W. Jarski et al., "A Comparison of Four Empathy Instruments in Simulated Patient–Medical Student Interactions," *Journal of Medical Education* 60 (1985): 545–551.

17. Holistic medicine, of course, should be the ideal medicine which takes care of the body as well as the soul. Unfortunately, the word holistic has been heavily abused by fringe groups who have jumped on the antimedical bandwagon. For the significance of this "holistic" medicine see A. S. Relman, "Holistic Medicine," *New England Journal of Medicine* 300 (1979): 312–313.

18. B. Inglis and R. West, *The Alternative Health Guide* (New York: Knopf, 1983).

19. Of one hundred patients who consulted physicians in one extensive study, about eighty-five suffered from a psychosocial problem or a self-limiting disease. L. P. Carmichael and J. S. Carmichael, "The Relational Model in Family Practice," in *Family Medicine: A New Approach to Health Care,* ed. B. E. Cogswell and M. B. Sussman (New York: Haworth Press, 1982), 123–133.

20. M. D. Altschule, "The Doctor-Patient Relationship through the Ages," *Alabama Journal of Medical Sciences* 21 (1984): 435–439.

21. I have weighed the *Index Medicus* for the year 1983 and came up with a figure of eighty pounds. This is bad enough, but fortunately well below the dire predictions of 1978, when D. T. Durack anticipated that the weight of the *Index Medicus* might reach a thousand kilograms by 1985; see "The Weight of Medical Knowledge," *New England Journal of Medicine* 298 (1978): 773–775.

22. M. R. Hawkins et al., "Sleep and Nutritional Deprivation and Performance of House Officers," *Journal of Medical Education* 605 (1985): 30–35.

23. R. S. Ulrich, "View through a Window May Influence Recovery from Surgery," *Science* 224 (1984): 420–421.

24. A. M. Harvey and V. A. McKusick, *Osler's Textbook Revisited* (New York: Appleton-Century-Crofts, 1967), 5–7.

# 11. *Thomas Merton the Healer*

**Robert Coles**

In the spring of 1955 I was an intern at the University of Chicago clinics. I had put in months of hard work in medicine and surgery. In February and March I had seen one patient after another die of leukemia and cancers that had eaten away their lungs, stomachs, and livers. I had worked day and night, trying to be of help to those patients, to the hospital's residents, to the attending physicians, to the medical students. A rough internship, all we interns consoled ourselves, but one that would last only a year. A particularly rough internship, we reminded ourselves with a touch of pride, as we mentioned the undeniable fact that, save a week's vacation, we never really could take for granted any time off. We could sign out, of course, but only if we were satisfied that we were not leaving any patients in jeopardy; that we'd done all the work that had to be done; and, not least, that we were "covered," meaning that another intern had agreed to take on our responsibilities, actual or potential, no matter his or her own evening or weekend obligations.

In my case such a request of another doctor was made difficult by my strenuous if not overwrought New England conscience. I was always afraid something terrible would take place in the middle of the night or on a Saturday or Sunday afternoon and that my absence would make a grim turn for the worse even grimmer: all those cards I carried, with all their medical information, would not be as readily usable in someone else's hands as they occasionally were in mine. Moreover, I wasn't then married, and so it was natural that those who were husbands or wives (one of us was the latter, among two women interns) would turn to a bachelor like me with a conviction, a willfulness I didn't seem able to muster with that question, Will you cover for me? Even if I knew how anxiously we all whistled in the dark, knew I'd likely as not be stuck with not one but two (or three or four) emergencies, perhaps a four-bell page (a patient dying then and there or, not rarely, found dead by a nurse) I still relented, thinking maybe, just maybe, the night would be quiet— four hours' sleep as opposed to none at all.

I summon those old days, those tough as hell days of a demanding internship because I want to describe an interlude which occurred in the midst of that year. My vacation took place in late March of 1955, and it followed a week of severe flu that had robbed me of energy and made me feel weak, tired, depressed, and, I regret to say, self-pitying. I kept wondering what I was doing, why I was where I was. I had stumbled into medicine, as it were. I got to know William Carlos Williams as a consequence of writing my undergraduate thesis on the first two books of *Paterson*, his long, lyrical evocation of America's complex social and cultural traditions; and then I became so enamored of him and his life (he was a hard-working physician as well as a writer) that I resolved to imitate that life, knowing full well I couldn't imitate his art. The result was a hasty (and not very successful) attempt to master premedical subjects and a lucky admission to Columbia University's College of Physicians and Surgeons, I suspect because the biochemist who interviewed me, Philip Miller (how well I remember that kindly man and the hour we spent together!) had read Williams' poems and short stories and novels and essays and didn't think me completely loony for trying to follow (partially at least) an admired other's lead. I had not done well at all in the first two years of medical school, and though I liked the last two years much better, I never did (as one doctor urged and warned me I must do) "get my act together." I was lucky, yet again, to get the relatively good university-connected internship I'd wanted—one in a hospital located wonderfully close to a college setting, I thought to myself so innocently as I left upon completion of a quick preliminary visit a few months before the end of medical school.

Now I was nearing the end of that internship hurdle, too, and I felt sadly lost as well as weary. I had no idea what I'd do next; I'd eliminated as possibilities most of the specialties because of my sense of inadequacy in relation to their requirements. Moreover, my body seemed ready to give out—not just a flu attack, but a cumulative exhaustion that seemed to be, at last, fearfully consuming. "You'd better *really* rest," I was told by Robert Ebert, then my "attending" (on the "medical chest service").

I knew my malaise wasn't only physical; I knew I was at loose ends about a career and I knew I had to do something to alter those circumstances. It never occurred to me to go see a psychiatrist nor had it then occurred to me to try to be one! I had read *The Seven Storey Mountain* by Thomas Merton in college at the urging of Perry Miller, my advisor at Harvard College, and for some reason had taken the book with me both to medical school and then to the hospital where I interned. As I struggled with the flu that spring and wondered what to do with or on my week of vacation, I found myself picking up Merton's book again and again. I even found myself realizing that Kentucky wasn't all that far from Illinois, and that Chicago wasn't a million miles from the spot where the Trappist monastery Gethsemani was located. (In it, as a day-to-day monk, lived Thomas Merton.)

The long and short of it was that I got into my car on the first morning of my week's respite, still coughing, throat sore, a fever of 100°, and headed south and then east. The next day, after a night in Louisville visiting a college friend, I headed nowhere in particular, as I'd told him, one minute thinking I'd end up in Cincinnati, visiting another college friend, the next minute thinking I'd just "bum around"—do a minor version of Kerouac, whose effort to comprehend and experience America Dr. W. C. Williams, himself quite old and ailing by then, had noted with interest and discussed with me several times in our phone conversations that past year.

But there were those other, odd moments; they had me looking intently at the map of Kentucky, remembering Merton's address. Eventually I showed up one late afternoon at the monastery he'd done so much, through his writing, to place in the consciousness of many fellow human beings. I drove through the adjoining farmland, past the wooded terrain, stopped my car in front of a modest (but to me, all of a sudden, fearfully imposing) building, reached for the door, turned the knob, noticed that there was no lock at work, and, soon enough, to condense things yet again, found myself a welcomed guest: I could stay, it seemed, as long as I wanted, though I had to understand the daily (and nightly) rhythms of those who had chosen to stay as long as life remained in their bodies.

Immediately upon entering the room given me and sitting on the bed to gather my thoughts, I realized that I both did, indeed, very much

want to see, meet, and talk with Thomas Merton—yet I had no right
to be where I was with such egotistic presumptions on my bedeviled
mind. I decided to leave the next day, but I also wanted to stay, to drink
up a particular haunting, unnerving atmosphere. This tourist's self-
indulgence, this self-serving thoughtlessness and arrogance, protected
me, I fear, all too well and in no way seemed to trouble those wise and
shrewdly observant monks, who had learned well to put up with the
likes of me, I later realized. By the time I had left that place in Kentucky
for good, two days later, I could say to myself that I'd met Thomas
Merton, that he had given me a warm smile, had made the sign of the
cross, had touched me in ways I didn't then understand and which, later,
when I'd become a psychiatrist and was in the middle of a prolonged
psychoanalysis, I'd try hard to figure out.

My analyst was not himself uninterested in religious matters, and as
we discussed that brief, increasingly clouded, obscure moment in my all
too lengthening life, I heard the word "healer" used: Merton as a healing writer, a healing presence. I wasn't sure what my analyst meant
when he used that descriptive category, but I knew I agreed with him,
with his use of it. More recently, I thought of that word "healer" as I
read Michael Mott's splendid biography of Merton and a recent volume
of selected letters Merton addressed to his many (oh, so many, and he
a cloistered monk) friends scattered all over the world. The biography
tells what Merton himself told in his celebrated autobiography and in
the many articles and books that followed it, an outpouring of passionate eloquence rendered readers throughout the world, in God's name, but
also, one dares say, and in no way to cast any skeptical shadows, out of
Merton's particular human calling as a healer. For he was one who began
knowing pain and watching suffering as an infant. His artist mother,
who austerely observed him when he was an infant and recorded her
daily impressions in a diary, became ill with cancer when he was scarcely
four years old, and when he was sixteen his father, also an artist, also
died of cancer. Lucky because he was born to parents of some standing
(talented, educated, not at all poor), he was thus unlucky, too. Even his
younger and only brother died young—killed in the Second World War
while fighting the Nazis. Merton lived a lonely if privileged youth, at-
tended private schools in England and then Columbia University in the
1930s, that "low dishonest decade," W. H. Auden called it, and all
the while tried to find his bearings: with the help of Freud and Marx;
through efforts to write journalism, poetry, fiction; by recourse to bouts
of drinking, sexual liaisons, intense spells of moody self-scrutiny; by
seeking lots of camaraderie and good food; and always by giving devoted attention to verse, to the stories of writers who had preceded him.

Finally there was the conversion to Catholicism and shortly thereafter the dedicated search for sanctity—the decision to give a lifetime to priestly contemplation and prayer as a Trappist. The irony is obvious— a man of letters, a man obsessed with words and their possibilities, chooses a monkhood which emphasizes silence and the strongest kind of self-abnegation. But there are additional ironies. Merton withdrew from the world when he entered the monastery, and yet he kept writing, pouring out his essays, poems, journal entries—one article after another, one book after another. The result was a worldwide following which included the famous and the utterly unknown. To all of his readers he gave consolation, advice, sympathy, understanding; he also offered ideas to consider, values to uphold. He was, of course, a Christian moralist, but he was also a bravely self-critical and confessional monk who dared to share his worries and hurts, his doubts and misgivings and fears with his correspondents, his readers. The power of *The Seven Storey Mountain,* of course, had to do with just that psychological candor, that willingness to be forthcoming on the part of a remarkably gifted lyrical writer. He was a craftsman of the English language who harnessed his literary skills to the task of an intense and continuing self-scrutiny and, yes, self-exposure. The result was a human being's suffering become redemptive—contagiously affecting others, prompting them to stop, think, wonder, ask questions, even take various moral or spiritual steps to follow Merton's healing lead, it may be said.

Dorothy Day and Daniel Berrigan and Walker Percy and so many others sought Merton out. I especially remember Dorothy Day's remarks about him: "He had known much pain, and he knew how to lift pain from others." She was content to state those two aspects of Merton without connecting the one to the other in what people like me call a psychodynamic way. Nevertheless, she knew that an essential and important part of Merton's life was his passionate desire to minister unto others, to hear from them, learn of their tensions and turmoils, and tell them of his, too. Once Dorothy Day said this about Merton as we talked of his voluminous writing: "He cured with words—all the time he did! I know! I can remember those letters, the good medicine that they were to me. And I always knew that with Merton it was the doctor healing himself as well as the rest of us who were his patients."

She was no stranger herself to such a healing effort, and her words about Merton echoed in my ears as I read the recent biography of him— a thoughtful inquiry aimed at comprehending an important life. The biographer is especially challenged by an anguished involvement Merton experienced late in life, one which stunned him, among others: the middle-aged monk, sick in the hospital, falls in love with his attending nurse. I have no desire here (or elsewhere) to probe psychologically or morally that time of passion and great apprehension and soul searching.

I simply want to point out that Merton had become a patient, and that a kind and generous nurse had surely reminded him of what he'd at least partially missed receiving as a child—the devoted, caring regard, the everyday healing of another person. But Merton the monk had found a way of redeeming his childhood losses. He followed the advice of St. Francis, he gave, and thereby received; he healed with poems and essays and letters and thereby himself was healed. But the healer suddenly vulnerable is the healer in great jeopardy, because exposed to the deepest sources of his or her calling, hence tempted yet again to try to redeem them, as that sick, bed-ridden monk endeavored to do: feel a deep and grateful love for the one attending him.

Not long afterward Merton would venture to Asia, ever anxious to be connected with wisdom and with healing other than the kind he knew. Yet while there he died suddenly, the victim of an accidental electrocution. A person present at the conference he had gone halfway across the world (Bangkok) to attend remarked upon his kindly manner, the gentleness he radiated and its calming effect on her: to the very last that humane touch of grace offered without guile or pretense to others.

# 12. *Words as Scalpels: Transmitting Evidence in the Clinical Dialogue*

Stanley J. Reiser

Throughout medical history physicians have pondered whether to discuss with patients the certainties and uncertainties about what is the matter and what might be done. Although the alternatives of disclosure or concealment have been forcefully argued for centuries, the problem remains nettlesome. A view of the ideas that have molded the shape of this issue over time may be helpful.

## Ancient and Medieval Medicine

Doctors who practiced in the Classical Age of Greek medicine worried about the risks of sharing knowledge with patients. In the Hippocratic writing "Decorum" the author cautions physicians to conceal "most things from the patient while you are attending him. Give orders with cheerfulness and serenity, turning his attention away from what is being done to him." The physician is told that many patients who learn of their condition or receive "a forecast of what is to come . . . [have] through this cause taken a turn for the worse."[1]

This statement reflects a viewpoint found in other places in the Hippocratic works. The doctor should take care not to upset the patient either by words or by other aspects of his person, such as bodily appearance ("he should look healthy, and as plump as nature intended him to be"), physiognomy ("let him be of a serious but not harsh countenance"), bearing ("he must be clean in person, well-dressed, and anointed with sweet-smelling unguents"), and character ("he must be grave and kind to all").[2] The physician must comfort the patient. Bad news, like rude behavior or uncomeliness, upsets the patient and is not appropriate as part of an acceptable bedside manner.

But what of the patient who is mortally ill? One Hippocratic writing, "Prorrhetikon II," counsels the physician to reveal the prognosis to a third person who, in turn, would tell the patient.[3] Some Greek works outside the Hippocratic corpus go even further in urging that those near death or suffering from illness likely to be chronic and debilitating learn about their prospects directly from the physician, and thus receive the undistorted facts needed to guide future actions. Whether patients decided to let nature determine the outcome or choose to end life through suicide (an acceptable alternative in Greek society), they would have had the opportunity to realize the social ideal of dying nobly—to bid farewell to family and friends, to face death squarely, to give death a place in life.[4]

The available literature suggests that in medieval times physicians often maintained a cheerful bearing before patients, made optimistic statements to them, and left to family and friends the task of giving bad news. The French surgeon Henri de Mondeville in the early fourteenth century advised colleagues to promise a cure to everyone whose case they decided to take, concealing disturbing news from them. But he suggested that relatives or friends get warning of danger, presumably to encourage patients to review secular affairs and receive, if necessary, last rites of the church. Surgical assistants were cautioned against discussing facts about the illness with patients unless the news was pleasant.[5] In another medieval treatise, attributed to Arnald of Villanova, doctors were urged to "promise health to the patient who is hanging on your lips" but to intentionally exaggerate the peril of the illness to the family. If the patient recovered, the physician was assured, "you will be praised more for your art; should he die his friends will testify that you had given him up."[6] No matter what the outcome, the doctor's reputation would be preserved.

## The Nineteenth Century

At the beginning of the nineteenth century, the general strategy of with-holding bad news from patients received a clear moral justification from the English physician Thomas Percival. It appeared in his most famous work, *Medical Ethics,* published in 1803 as a guide to appropriate con-duct for doctors in relations with professional colleagues and patients. In one section headed "A Physician should be the minister of hope and comfort to the sick," after citing conflicting arguments by several philoso-phers and physicians on the subject, Percival declared his position. The right of patients to know the truth "is suspended, and even annihilated" if it would prove damaging to them, their family, or the community. The expectation of patients to be shielded by doctors from harm required it. In cases producing a conflict between the physician's "delicate sense of ve-racity, which is so ornamental to, and indeed forms a characteristic excel-lence of, the virtuous man, [and the] claim of Professional justice and social duty" that bound the doctor to protect the patient from injury, "a wise and good man must be governed by those which are the most im-perious; and will therefore generously relinquish every consideration re-ferable only to himself." Still, Percival cautioned the doctor "not to do this, but in cases of real emergency, which happily seldom occur; and to guard his mind sedulously against the injury it may sustain by such vio-lations of the native love of truth." [7]

Percival's position on truth telling was adopted by many physicians in the nineteenth century. The code of medical ethics proposed at the found-ing meeting of the American Medical Association in 1846 and published in 1847 discloses an acceptance of Percival's recommendations as well as a continuity with attitudes expressed in the ancient Greek and medi-eval periods.

> A physician should not be forward to make gloomy prognostica-tions, because they savour of empiricism, by magnifying the im-portance of his services in the treatment or cure of the disease. But he should not fail, on proper occasions, to give to the friends of the patient timely notice of danger, when it really occurs; and even to the patient himself, if absolutely necessary. This office, however, is so peculiarly alarming when executed by him, that it ought to be declined whenever it can be assigned to any other person of suffi-cient judgment and delicacy. For, the physician should be the min-ister of hope and comfort to the sick; that, by such cordials to the drooping spirit, he may smooth the bed of death, revive expiring life, and counteract the depressing influence of those maladies which often disturb the tranquility of the most resigned in their last

moments. The life of a sick person can be shortened not only by the acts, but also by the words or the manner of a physician. It is, therefore, a sacred duty to guard himself carefully in this respect, and to avoid all things which have a tendency to discourage the patient and to depress his spirits.[8]

These views were ratified in the second half of the nineteenth century by leading figures in American medicine. Austin Flint, the New York practitioner, warned that "undue solemnity, anxiety, and apprehension in the looks, manner or words" of a doctor discouraged patients, while "a cheerful mien, calmness of deportment, and verbal assurances" often accomplished more than drugs.[9] If there was danger of error, Flint thought it was far better to err by looking on the bright side.

In this position Flint was joined by Harvard professor of anatomy Oliver Wendell Holmes: "Your patient has no more right to all the truth you know than he has to all the medicine in your saddlebags. . . . He should get only as much as is good for him." Holmes emphasized the gravity of depriving patients of hope. He cautioned physicians against betraying their apprehensions by looks: "The face of a physician like that of a diplomatist should be impenetrable." He also urged doctors to be very careful about the medical terms they used: a patient might know their meaning or consult a dictionary. Yet for patients who insisted on learning what disease they had but were without apparent capacity to understand a scientific explanation, Holmes remarked that "shrewd old doctors have a few phrases always on hand." Holmes found the term "spinal irritation" to serve him well on some occasions. Still, he thought "nothing on the whole has covered so much ground, and meant so little, and given such profound satisfaction to all parties, as the magnificent phrase 'congestion of the portal system.'"[10]

Views on truth telling were usually transmitted to medical students by example rather than precept; it was uncommon for professors to explicitly discuss the subject. Richard Cabot, while a medical student at the end of the nineteenth century, recalls it addressed only once during his education: "'When you are thinking of telling a lie,' said one of his teachers, 'ask yourself whether it is simply and solely for the patient's benefit that you are going to tell it. If you are sure that you are acting for his good and not for your own profit, you can go ahead with a clear conscience.'"[11]

## The Twentieth Century

Many twentieth-century physicians treated this issue as their nineteenth-century predecessors did. In a 1927 article for a popular magazine, a physician recommended that medical practitioners skillfully mix "false-hood and truth in order to provide the patient with an amalgam which will make the metal of life wear and keep men from being . . . unpleas-ing to themselves and to those who love them." [12] His view was deter-mined by the uncertainties of predicting prolonged illness or death, the possibility that a cure for the condition in question could materialize in the future, and the seeming reluctance of patients to receive anxiety-provoking news about their health.

Practitioners of this period in their approach to truth telling seemed to be following a precept of medicine enunciated in the Hippocratic work "Epidemics I" "to at least do no harm." [13] Harvard biochemist and phy-sician L. J. Henderson in 1935 specifically cited this advice in caution-ing colleagues that they could inflict damage on patients by lying and by truth telling as well. "Try to do as little harm as possible, not only in treatment with drugs, or with the knife, but also in treatment with words." [14] Similar sentiments were expressed in a 1955 collection of es-says in which well-known physicians discussed the question, Should the patient know the truth? Most agreed with the book's editor, who an-swered yes if the knowledge of the truth improved the patient's prospects of recovery, no if it diminished them. [15]

"No problem is more vexing than the decision about what to tell the cancer patient," wrote Chicago psychiatrist Donald Oken in his 1961 survey on physicians' behavior after diagnosing cancer. [16] Of the some two-hundred doctors he questioned, almost 90 percent usually withheld diagnoses from patients. Their basic attitude was to tell "as little as pos-sible in the most general terms consistent with maintaining cooperation in treatment." Questions raised by patients were usually disregarded and treated as pleas for reassurance, unless persistent. Most of the physi-cians believed that virtually all patients did not want to know they had cancer, that justification was required for disclosing the truth, not for withholding it. For all physicians queried, the most important goal of their actions—whether patients were told about their diagnosis or not—was the maintenance of hope. "Every single physician interviewed spon-taneously emphasized this point. . . . Each in his own way communi-cates the possibility, even the likelihood, of recovery." In forming their policy toward truth telling, factors such as illness in friends or family were cited as relatively minor determinants, with medical education listed by only eleven respondents as having any bearing on their be-havior. (Few recalled the subject discussed in their training, and when they did could not remember what was said other than it had been ad-dressed.) Most cited clinical experience as the central element in deter-mining their position. Yet exploration of this point in later interviews made this explanation doubtful. Only 14 percent had ever tried any approach to truth telling other than the one they currently used. Further, most could not remember instances in which approaches different from their own had unfavorable consequences—indeed those they knew of had satisfactory outcomes. "Instead of logic and rational decision based on critical observation," wrote Oken, "what is found is opinion, belief, and conviction, heavily weighted with emotional justification."

Another examination of doctors' attitudes toward disclosure came from physicians John Stoeckle and Howard Waitzkin in 1972. They pointed to studies showing that doctors often withheld diagnoses and prognoses not only from mortally ill patients but also from those whose lives were not necessarily threatened—patients with poliomyelitis or tuberculosis. These results implied doctors managed clinical evidence in a way that tended to maintain authority: *"A physician's ability to preserve his own power over the patient in the doctor-patient relationship depends largely on his ability to control the patient's uncertainty"* about the course of the illness, the nature of therapy, and the physician's future actions.[17] To the investigators this postulated association of power and uncertainty accounted for the doctor's particular hesitancy in revealing a prognosis to a dying patient; to do so was a declaration of powerlessness, a confession that the doctor's technical ability could not overcome the problem.

## Arguments for Disclosure

An early plea against benevolent deception in explanations about illness is found in *A Discourse upon the Duties of a Physician* written by Samuel Bard, an American physician, and published in 1769. He was concerned about the possible damaging influence of bad news to a patient: "Shew your Apprehension of his Danger, rather by your Assiduity to relieve, than by any harsh or brutal Expressions of it." Yet Bard was unyielding in his counsel about the dying patient. "Never buoy up a dying Man with groundless Expectations of Recovery." At best it was well-intended deception, at worst it was a means of extracting more money from the patient for additional medical care. Withholding such information was also pointless. He believed that by meditation, philosophical reasoning, and religion "the grim Tyrant may in general be disarmed of his Terrors, and rendered familiar to the most timid, and apprehensive."[18] Explaining the facts was kinder and wiser than concealing them.

A more comprehensive argument favoring disclosure in the medical relationship was written nearly a century later in 1849 by American physician Worthington Hooker.[19] In part, it was a response to arguments made by Thomas Percival. Hooker disputed the assertion, upon which the policy of concealment was usually based, that bad news inevitably harmed patients. The experience of physicians who pursued a candid course with patients contradicted this orthodox view. He challenged the belief that efforts at concealment generally succeeded. An unguarded hint by those who were colluding, an innocent remark by some who were not, usually revealed to the patient the true state of things and produced a reaction far worse than could be imagined had candor been used from the start. The patient's initial dismay and resentment was frequently followed by profound suspicion and doubt of everything said about the illness. Moreover, the effects of the deception usually spread beyond the patient deceived. It damaged the general confidence of people in the veracity of physicians and undermined the efforts of doctors in medical situations where belief in the doctor's veracity was crucial to a patient's recovery. There was also the danger that physicians would become habituated to deception—small untruths making larger ones increasingly easy to perpetrate. Hooker further argued, as Kant had earlier in his treatise *On a Supposed Right to Tell Lies from Benevolent Motives,* that although one could never know the unintended and cumulative effects of a deception, the instigator was morally liable for all of them. The sacrifice of truth in pursuit of some higher end tragically resulted in the sacrifice of this greatest good, this aspect of behaving that underlay all relations in a moral universe. What, then, did Hooker suggest as policy for the communication of information in the medical relationship? He acknowledged the need to sometimes conceal facts from the sick that might be injurious to them. But he insisted that in withholding the truth no deception be used, no falsehood be put in its place.

Arguments of the sort made by Hooker are expressed at the beginning of the twentieth century by Richard Cabot. An experience early in his medical career was decisive in forming his attitude. While making an effort to conceal the truth about a patient's illness from his wife, she challenged him to answer honestly every question she asked. He halted the ruse, and the expected harms failed to occur. This prompted him to experiment gingerly with telling the truth in cases such as this one where, apparently, it could not be borne by the parties involved. Cabot was surprised by the "astounding *innocuousness of the truth* when all reason and all experience would lead one to believe it must do harm. . . . No one ought to believe this who has not tried it," he declared. Cabot did not suggest that physicians explore the minutest details and contingencies of illness with a patient; his was not a call for the "naked truth" that might confuse or frighten patients. Rather, Cabot urged physicians to give the patient a "true impression" of the illness, a portrait describing not only the dangers and limitations to life but also the possibilities for remission and the prospects for enjoyment that the illness

would likely allow. Yet he appreciated that such explanations were difficult and time consuming; that because of this physicians were inclined
to "give the patient either a rough half-truth or a smooth lie." [20]

Cabot's emphasis on the skillful exercise of clinical method in re-
laying painful information to patients appears in the work of Cicely
Saunders in England and Elisabeth Kübler-Ross in the United States
which gained attention in the 1960s. Saunders argues that all patients,
curable or incurable, need their illnesses explained and interpreted to
them in a convincing manner. This relieves their fears and allows them
to cooperate most fully with their physician in therapy. She calls attention to the importance of nonverbal communication in doctor-patient relationships—the gaps, silences, and facial expressions that often say
more than words. She urges physicians to give patients time to come to
grips with their feelings and thoughts about the illness and to bear in
mind what for her is the key therapeutic question, "What do you let
your patients tell you?" [21] Saunders' principal argument against a policy
that involves a consistent denial of unpleasant facts is the difficulty it in-
troduces into communications between doctor and patient. Kübler-Ross
in her emphasis on method in communication with patients touches on
many of the issues that Saunders does. [22] But she places greater stress on
the need of physicians to understand their own attitudes toward suffering
and dying in order to deal with those feelings in patients.

## Shifts in Attitudes

In the 1970s a candid approach to giving clinical information was urged
by scholars in ethics and philosophy such as Sissela Bok: "The goal
must be disclosure, and the atmosphere one of openness." [23] Growing
numbers of laymen answered the call. Surveys indicated that despite
their fears, even when confronted with a life-threatening illness such as
cancer, most people, both the well and the sick, desired to know the diagnosis and prognosis and felt helped more than harmed by the news. [24]
Although a majority of patients may have held this view before, it was
becoming increasingly well documented.

The attitudes of doctors underwent revision at this time. A study conducted in 1977 which asked a group of physicians the same questions
Oken had in 1961 revealed sharp alterations in behavior. [25] Of the 264
respondents, 98 percent affirmed the value of being totally frank with
patients who have cancer. Although medical school teaching and hospital training now had a greater influence on attitudes toward information
giving, for most physicians in the new study, as in the older one, unexamined conviction rather than rational study basically determined their

position. Of further interest, 100 percent of the responding doctors, compared with 60 percent in the 1961 survey, said they would want to be told if they had cancer. And all of the doctors queried in 1977 affirmed the patient's right to know the diagnosis.

Some causes of this attitudinal change appear to be improved therapy for cancer, giving physicians more to offer patients and allowing patients to be more optimistic about cure and willing to hear about their condition; increased fear of malpractice suits, encouraging doctors to diminish legal liability by more fully informing patients; a better understanding by physicians of the dying process; legal requirements to disclose diagnoses to patients in experimental protocols; and studies indicating that many of the doctors' anxieties about giving patients bad news are groundless.[26] Perhaps most crucial is an alteration of social opinion about the right of patients to medical truth.

This alteration, which has affected disclosure of clinical data in all aspects of medicine, became influential in the mid 1960s. Then government-mandated human studies committees were established at all medical institutions conducting federally sponsored research. They regulated the process of informing subjects about the risks and benefits of experiments in which they were asked to participate. Such directed attention to the right of patients to learn the risks of experimental interventions spread to clinical practice. In 1973 the American Hospital Association issued a twelve-point "Patient's Bill of Rights."[27] It specified many aspects of therapy the patient should know of and the doctor should reveal.

Strong pressures on the side of disclosure from groups outside of and within medicine have continued to mount. Just recently, for example, a panel of experts was convened by the National Institutes of Health to examine the controversial question of whether to use estrogens to treat menopausal symptoms. They could make no technical recommendation suitable for all patients and suggested that the decision to use estrogens should hinge on a joint discussion and appraisal of risks and benefits by doctor and patient. The panel urged doctors to give patients "as much information as possible about the evidence for the effectiveness of estrogens in treating specific menopausal conditions and the risks of their use" and also to keep them "continually informed of new findings as they arise."[28]

Such insistence on bringing patients into the process of clinical decision making will probably grow in the future, affecting the care not only of those with life-threatening diseases but also the care of all patients and every aspect of the therapeutic encounter.

## The Contemporary Physician

The historical record indicates physicians have recognized that words can wound as deeply as knives, that what is said can be as significant as what is done. Those who argue that disclosure of threatening news should be the rule instead of the exception bear weighty burdens. They must have prepared themselves to learn spoken and silent cues patients telegraph about facts they know or crave about their illnesses, to communicate effectively with patients and sustain them emotionally once the news is out, to understand psychological difficulties that can accompany disclosure, and to allocate time for the often lengthy period over which disclosure can take place. They must also recognize that the harms created by inadequate mastery of the techniques and skills of communicating bad news may outweigh the benefits of the individual of learning the truth.

Physicians who believe threatening news should be generally withheld from patients, or who yield to the pressures of families to adopt this course, face equally difficult problems. They must justify abridging a widely held social and moral expectation that veracity should govern doctor-patient relationships, deal with the quandaries of treating patients without giving them explanations that satisfactorily justify therapeutic actions, and worry about the effects on the illness that hearsay evidence acquired by patients may have, as well as possible harm borne by patients unable to penetrate an isolating wall of hopeful or equivocal statements to discuss forebodings, to say or do things that knowledge of future prospects would allow. Physicians supporting this view must also be regardful of the considerable stress their decision to withhold diagnoses or prognoses can place on other members of the hospital staff (such as nurses, clergy, students) and on families, all of whom must deal with the patient's anxieties and questions but usually without adequate clinical insight about the course of the illness or clear authority to assume the physician's responsibility for deciding what to disclose.

This subject generates a considerable emotional response in medicine that often obscures a distinction, central to the wise use of clinical knowledge, between withholding opinions while in the process of deciding and discussing conclusions after evaluation has been completed. There is no basic medical or moral reason to explore contingencies with patients on the way to reaching clinical judgments. The appropriate time for sharing diagnostic information with them is after the physician has arrived at some conclusion about its significance. This does not mean the doctor must be sure about what the illness is or its outcome, but that a point has been reached in the process of clinical study where further investigation either will not resolve uncertainties or will not overturn seemingly well-founded evidence. Then, in my view, discussion of the findings with the patient is warranted but not an extensive scientific discussion of minute details, remote contingencies, and difficult judgments about conflicting data, what one doctor might tell another. What is called for, as Richard Cabot suggested a half-century ago, is a "true impression" that, in terms understood by the patient, broadly outlines the doctor's conclusions and presents them in a way that minimizes despair, sustains self-worth, and heeds cues from the patient in setting the pace of disclosure.

The method of informing and its timing are crucial. Yet here many physicians encounter problems. Much of medical education is devoted to learning how to gather and evaluate facts, little to how to divulge them. And to divulge unskillfully and uncritically is to court inflicting grievous harms on patients.

If medical educators more explicitly explored with students the origins of their emotional and intellectual attitudes toward giving and receiving bad news and took advantage of modern knowledge about communication and interviewing, they could help students develop greater ability to discuss threatening events with patients and at the same time free them from the foreboding anxiety of causing harm that restrained their predecessors. Current writing about the moral dimensions of the medical relationship and techniques of applying principles of ethics to clinical problems also provide new opportunities to recognize, understand, and resolve the ethical dilemmas of giving and keeping evidence. These possibilities suggest that perhaps we will find that good clinical method and disclosure are not the antagonistic pair that generations of doctors have considered them.

Still it remains a gray area of clinical and ethical judgment of how best to handle news that could be alarming to patients: more must be learned, and moralizing avoided. Enough work has been done, however, to provide at least a broad picture of some important problems that accompany the matter. As in many aspects of medical life, the physician must choose, and act, before all the facts are in.

## Notes

1. Hippocrates, "Decorum," in W. H. S. Jones, trans., *Hippocrates,* vol. 2 (Cambridge, Mass.: Harvard University Press, 1923), 297.

2. Hippocrates, "The Physician," in ibid., 311, 313.

3. L. Edelstein, "Hippocratic Prognosis," in O. Temkin and C. L. Temkin, eds., *Ancient Medicine: Selected Papers of Ludwig Edelstein* (Baltimore: Johns Hopkins University Press, 1967), 76.

4. Edelstein, "Hellenism of Greek Medicine," in ibid., 384.

5. D. Power, ed., *Treatises of Fistula in Ano* (London: Kegan, Paul, Trench, Trubner and Co., 1910), xx.

6. Arnald of Villanova (?), "De cautelis medicorum," in H. E. Sigerist, trans., *Bulletin of the Northwest University Medical School* 20 (1946): 139–142.

7. T. Percival, *Medical Ethics,* 3rd ed. (Oxford: John Henry Parker, 1849), 140.

8. American Medical Association, "First Code of Medical Ethics," in *Proceedings of the National Medical Convention 1846–1847* (Chicago: American Medical Association, 1847), 94.

9. A. Flint, "Medical Ethics and Etiquette," *New York Medical Journal* 37 (1883): 340–345.

10. O. W. Holmes, "The Young Practitioner," in *Medical Essays* (Boston: Houghton Mifflin, 1883), 388.

11. R. C. Cabot, "The Use of Truth and Falsehood in Medicine: An Experimental Study," *American Medicine* 5 (1903): 344–349.

12. J. Collins, "Should Doctors Tell the Truth?" *Harper's Monthly Magazine* 155 (1927): 320–326.

13. See Jones, *Hippocrates,* vol. 1, 165.

14. L. J. Henderson, "Physician and Patient as a Social System," *New England Journal of Medicine* 212 (1935): 819–823.

15. S. Standard and H. Nathan, eds., *Should the Patient Know the Truth?* (New York: Springer Publishing Co., 1955), 18.

16. D. Oken, "What to Tell Cancer Patients: A Study of Medical Attitudes," *Journal of the American Medical Association* 175 (1961): 1120–1128.

17. H. Waitzkin and J. D. Stoeckle, "The Communication of Information about Illness," *Advanced Psychosomatic Medicine* 8 (1972): 185–189, my italics.

18. S. Bard, *A Discourse upon the Duties of a Physician* (New York: A. and J. Robertson, 1769), 10.

19. W. Hooker, *Physician and Patient* (New York: Baker and Scribner, 1849), 357–382.

20. Cabot, "Use of Truth and Falsehood," my italics.

21. C. M. S. Saunders, "Telling Patients," *District Nursing* (September 1965): 149–150, 154.

22. E. Kübler-Ross, *On Death and Dying* (New York: Macmillan, 1970).

23. S. Bok, *Lying: Moral Choice in Public and Private Life* (New York: Pantheon Books, 1978), 239.

24. "Should Dying Patients Be Told the Truth?" *MGH News* 38, no. 2 (1979): 7–8; M. Blumenfield, N. B. Levy, and D. Kaufman, "Do Patients Want to Be Told?" *New England Journal of Medicine* 299 (1978): 1138; Kübler-Ross, *On Death and Dying,* 229.

25. D. H. Novack, E. J. Freireich, and S. Vaisrub, "Changes in Physicians' Attitudes toward Telling the Cancer Patient," *Journal of the American Medical Association* 241 (1979): 897–900.

26. Ibid.; E. J. Freireich, "Should the Patient Know?" *Journal of the American Medical Association* 241 (1979): 928.

27. American Hospital Association, "Statement on a Patient's Bill of Rights," *Hospitals* 47 (1973): 41.

28. National Institute on Aging, National Institutes of Health, "Estrogen Use and Postmenopausal Women: A National Institutes of Health Consensus Development Conference," *Annual Internal Medicine* 91 (1979): 921–922.

# 13. *Placebos, Patients, and Physicians*

Howard M. Spiro

The placebo stands at the center of the conflict between science and intuition, reminding physicians that science alone may not be sufficient for medical practice. Contemplation of the placebo reminds us physicians of so much of what we do *not* know. During the 1982–83 academic year I was a fellow at the Center for Advanced Study in the Behavioral Sciences at Stanford, California, reading and reflecting about my thirty-five years as a physician. I thought about the models of medicine, the metaphors by which we physicians fashion our lives and evaluate our tasks, and came to doubt whether the metaphors of physician as fighter against death or as scientist and detective are sufficient. I have concluded that for me, at least, they are not.

While at the center I audited a course in contract law at Stanford Law School. I was curious to see how law students were trained, what our fellow professionals learned and how. Also, because there is so much talk about "contract" and "covenant" in medical ethics, I wanted to learn firsthand what lawyers mean by contract. Of the many contrasts I

saw between medical school and law school, one struck me the most
forcibly. In their search for fairness and justice, lawyers—and judges—
recognize that the law creates only a temporary "truth," that "up there"
in Plato's sky there is no truth that they will uncover. Many lawyers see
the law as serving social purposes; they understand that decisions turned
one way at one time will be reversed at another. Law school teaching
seems to be, in a phrase, divergent—many different opinions are not
only possible but plausible. In the contract law course, at least, law students learn to look at problems from every possible angle, and after they
have exhausted every possibility the instructor suggests, "Well, suppos-
ing we change things a little bit . . . what then?" And the discussion
goes on. Sometimes a bit sophistic to the medical observer accustomed
to the search for facts, law school teaching provides a sharp contrast to
medical training as I have watched it.

For physicians, I think, whether in medical research or in practice,
Truth is always being uncovered or discovered. The lawyers teach and
understand divergence; but in medical theory and practice, so it seems
to me, we teach and believe in convergence. All of us, physicians, medical students, and research scientists, are scratching away tryng to uncover the one truth. We teach algorithms as one way to the diagnosis and
indeed sometimes the only way. Looking to molecular biology for all the
answers to disease suggests less rather than more diversity. To be sure,
molecular biology and technological development have revolutionized
beyond the dreams of thirty years ago what physicians can do, but my
experiences at Yale and Stanford law schools have made me wonder
whether physicians who take care of the sick should not open themselves to the unknown rather than insist only on the known and the
quantifiable.

I have been looking at the placebo, because I have been looking back
at my three decades or so as a gastroenterologist. The increasing number of practicing gastroenterologists in Connecticut over the past three
decades has very much changed my activities as a consultant. I see
many patients with abdominal pain that has not been explained by the
legions of imaging studies, and it is those patients with pain who have
intrigued me the most and who have frustrated me the most often. I do
not know why they have their pain, and I am not always able to relieve
it. Moreover, when I observe in controlled clinical trials how physio-
logically inactive agents can bring profound relief of ulcer pain (which
tells me that the physician is more than a mere conveyor of power and
pills and technology), I find myself wondering at the power of the
placebo.

Look at the clinical drama of placebos. A physician gives a patient
with a complaint an inactive pill, and the patient's complaints are re-

lieved, to a greater or lesser extent. How much that sequence can tell us, and yet how little has been written and how little is said in everyday teaching about the placebo. To be found reading about the placebo in a library, at least in California, is like being found in a pornographic bookstore. When I tell my friends that I find much to praise about the placebo, in pity they comment that I have "gone Californian." Yet although I have found much that is written and accepted about the placebo to be an exaggeration or a misinterpretation of observations, I have also found contemplation of the placebo to be a good way to focus on the conflict between science and intuition in medical practice.

That conflict is a real one. It looked as if science was all that was necessary for modern medicine, but the prevalence in our society of hosts of holistic practitioners suggests that contemplating the unmeasurable may still have something to offer. In their too rare moments of contemplation, most physicians see themselves, at least in their younger years, as scientists and heirs of the Enlightenment, that remarkable period in the eighteenth century when reason, natural science, and faith in progress all seemed to be coming together to move culture and society ever onward and upward. In the United States, particularly, the heirs of Jefferson and Franklin, the Unitarians and the transcendentalists, continue to believe that progress is inevitable. The modern physician seems to have little patience for the idea of the pendulum and the notion that opinions may swing back and forth. We have good reason for optimism. From the triumphs of antibiotics against infectious diseases, which began about forty years ago, to the harnessing of bacteria to our will, scientific achievement has advanced ever more rapidly and has changed the tasks and lives of physicians dramatically. Who would ever have thought that bacteria like *E. coli* would be slaving away to produce interferon, that genes could be moved or plucked out or polished up? Surely physicians can be forgiven for thinking that the scientific method would provide solutions to all diseases. Many optimists, indeed, agree that finding the right gene or the right switch to turn on or off will make most human diseases disappear and maybe we shall all live to be 120 or more.

It is hard for me to share that halcyon view. One disease always seems to replace another. If one bacterial species retreats, to continue the military motif so popular in talking about diseases, another advances in its place. Gastroenterologists have rejoiced at the decline in frequency of peptic ulcer, in large part recently owing to the $H_2$ blockers, but peptic ulcer was slowly decreasing in frequency before the advent of cimetidine. Regardless, we see fewer patients with peptic ulcer but many more with Crohn's disease; fewer patients with cancer of the stomach, but cancer of the pancreas has taken its place. I do not think that we physicians should conclude that our work will soon be taken from us or that we shall spend our declining years dealing only with the results of trauma.

Medical history, with only a few exceptions, is written, at least by physicians, as if medical practice were isolated from its enveloping social and intellectual culture and from historical trends. In many ways, reading medical history is much like reading Genesis; you want to skip over all the "begats." Hebrew names may be replaced in large part by European ones, but medical history until very recently focused on medical personages and discoveries more than on the mainstream of intellectual and scientific thought, which so influences what physicians do and think. The overemphasis on method, on fact, and on quantification is not unique to medicine but stems from the eighteenth-century period of Enlightenment. While we can trace the conflict between science and intuition all the way back to Hippocratic writers, who believed in empiricism and observation, and to Aesculapius, who stood for the magical qualities of medical practice, still modern medical science descends directly from the eighteenth- and nineteenth-century scientific traditions.

Yet we physicians live in two worlds: the world of science, which provides us with our ideals and with the real advances against diseases, and the world of people, persons with instincts, with pain, suffering, hope, and joy. We have a hard time separating out what we learn in science from what we need in practice to deal with people. The placebo reminds us to focus on the interface between those two worlds.

The scientific method is responsible for the only real advances in the understanding of disease; but house officers particularly need to be reminded that although science builds the steps of the ladder of progress, science is not, at least at present, sufficient to answer all human needs in medicine. They treat sick patients with acute diseases, with acute exacerbation of chronic problems, in an acute hospital setting. Beset by the need to learn technical skills, they seem to have little time for people as such, for the patient with the disease; I fear they grow impatient with those around them who cannot add to their fund of facts, or techniques, or list of recent references. Some of the more contemplative ones wonder if medical practice for the rest of their lives will be only dealing with "train wrecks," and some more humanistically oriented may even wonder whether they made the right decision—to study medicine.

House officers find some liquid surcease at the Friday afternoon colloquia at my hospital, known as "open library," but other refreshment might be even more restorative. Anthropology, history, literature, and poetry have as much to teach physicians about what they do not know as science does about what they should know. In the medieval colleges, courses were divided between the *trivium,* with its emphasis on the verbal topics of grammar, rhetoric, and logic, and the *quadrivium,* the measuring sciences of mathematics, geometry, astronomy, and music. Over the past few generations medical teaching has emphasized the quadrivial and has relegated the trivial to the later years, after the residency and in clinical practice. More emphasis on the trivial in the residency years would be helpful.

Why is the importance of the humanities in medicine so much talked about and so long complimented at graduation exercises, and why has so little changed in the curriculum? It may be partly because medical school has become the training time for house officers and not for practicing physicians. It may also be because there are no examinations in the medical school in the humanities, partly because few powerful forces—whether professors or foundations—sponsor humanities in medicine at our medical schools, and finally because those who talk about the nonmeasurable in the medical schools are seen as failed scientists, as abortive scientists, even hollow individuals, if you like. The emphasis in medical training is on quantification, on what can be measured, and few are interested in the placebo response because it is so hard to find something to measure.

Yet as I have said, the placebo reminds us of the interface at which we physicians live. A placebo has been defined as any therapy deliberately used by a physician for its nonspecific psychological effect. A physician gives what he or she believes to be an inert material to a sick person with a complaint, which may or may not be from a detectable disease, and after that the complaint is lessened. Physicians may give a placebo as a gift, to relieve a pain or to treat a complaint in a benevolent mode; a challenge, to prove to patients that their complaints have "no organic origin"; or a ransom, to get demanding or difficult patients out of their office. I shall not now review placebo effects, except to tell you that from my reading I believe that the only thing that the placebo relieves is pain, anxiety, or suffering. I have examined most of the other reported evidence, and I find nothing to convince me that a disease itself is remarkably changed, for better or worse, by a placebo. The placebo treats the patient, not the disease—improves the "functional" aspects of disease, if you will. But the relief of pain that comes to patients is a useful reminder of how much more than disease and sickness, the objective structural change we all try to detect, is pain and suffering, the experience of illness.

My reading has convinced me that the placebo should be used only in the benevolent mode, when it functions as a symbol, in some way to stimulate the internal healing powers of the patient. These healing powers, so much talked about in the lay and even professional literature, are largely directed at the perception of pain and its attendant affective states of anxiety, apprehension, and the like, but that is no mean target. I may think that receiving a placebo and having faith in it stimulates my endorphins or raises my gate threshold for the perception of pain, I may find a physiological explanation in raised endorphin levels or in an effect on cortical mechanisms in the brain, but the mechanism itself is not really the important point for physicians. To a large extent, truth has passed from what the patient perceives, so far as the physician is concerned, to what the physician can find. But if patients tell their physicians that their pain is less or that they feel better, discovery of a mechanism by which that report can be objectified should not make the report in itself any more or less meaningful.

Does the mechanism matter? Surely, someday how a placebo works will be clear and may even be quantified. At the moment, however, clinicians are much like the traveler in the desert who finds a stone buried in the dust. He brushes the sand off the stone and finds some hieroglyphics. He has found evidence that some person worked on the stone to leave a message, but he cannot read the message. When I read in *Science* that memory, in the mollusk at least, may depend upon the calcium channels and calmodulin, I was intrigued. But I remind myself that brain events are not mind events, and at least for the foreseeable future even working out the circuits of the brain will not tell me where gratitude may be found, or where hope or love join together in the pathways of the brain. I conclude that for the present it is enough to accept the report that pain is relieved by a placebo, and I do not worry too much about the mechanism.

Should physicians use a placebo for some patients? I think so, but there are some well-known dangers, for physicians who use them may delude themselves into thinking that their patient has no significant organic disease because the placebo relieves the patient's pain; find the placebo a first step to more major deceit or diagnostic ennui; or mistakenly believe that the placebo response indicates that the complaint is feigned.

Placebos relieve pain, how often I am not sure. In peptic ulcer studies pain is relieved, let us say, 60 percent of the time, but I am not sure how far I can extend that figure. How placebos work demands further study and contemplation. Whom they work upon is equally vague. There seems to be no specific personality types that can be predicted by any criterion to be more or less susceptible to the placebo response. Much has been ventured in this area, but little has emerged.

Some physicians, particularly in our scientific era, refuse even to consider using a placebo and look on those who do as not very different from witch doctors or voodoo healers. Trained to be rational scientists, they feel that they have professional responsibilities to maintain and their integrity to think about. They are right, to some extent. No physi-

cian should suspend his or her rational judgment. Reports of the benefit of placebo must be weighed in the same balance as reports of the
efficacy of any new drug or any new controlled clinical trial. Methods
must be reasonable; some methods are going to prove more reliable than
others, and many accounts of the placebo effect are unsound. I do not
accept all anecdotal experiences as generalizable or all reports as equally
valid. I simply am suggesting that physicians should begin to evaluate
such reports, to take another look at the placebo, and try to put its use
into some kind of context or pattern.

For the placebo has many good lessons for me as a physician. It
teaches me that disease and illness are both somewhat different matters.
We need to talk about how a disease differs from an illness, what we
mean by patients and persons, and how furiously health must be pursued. We need to have discussions about these issues, to learn that pain
and suffering are as important to the patient as whether he or she has
a disease that we can see or not. In many ways contemplation of the
placebo and how and when it works may help the physician move from
the biomechanical-biomedical model as sufficient for all disease and illness (if not for all human complaints) to a model that takes into account
the social, personal, psychological, and cultural implications of getting
sick.

What the placebo does, I think, is tell the patient that he or she has a
connection, that some person, a physician, I hope, is going to try to
help. Maybe all it does is speed up the transference reaction, but then
the countertransference may be equally important. Giving a placebo in
the right mode does something for the physician, too. It makes him or
her recognize that there is a patient "out there," that there is someone
beyond the image of the plastic card, that the icon of disease stands for a
person.

Let me repeat that what the placebo does is to act as the symbol of a
connection—tangible evidence that some person cares and will try to do
something. How that knowledge then relieves pain or anxiety I do not
now know; but the rational scientific physician should not be ashamed to
throw out the lifeline. Again, the placebo reminds us that we are dealing
with living patients, that we must listen, that we must engage in a dialogue. More than just looking at a disease, we must hear our patients.

The placebo has many other lessons to teach. It emphasizes the difference between the eye and the ear in medical diagnosis. Over the past
years, as physicians have come to depend upon imaging techniques to
show them disease, they have lost faith in simply hearing about the complaints from the patients. Complaints are evanescent, to the physician at
least; they are words uttered, listened to, that "float away on the air," in
Ong's lovely phrase. Only the image is real, whether on X-ray, echo, or

endoscopic film; disease as an image is abstracted, flattened, given a reality that makes it seem more important than the patient, who fades into the background. Images freeze the idea of disease and encourage physician-to-physician communication rather than physician-to-patient conversation. Images denature and dehumanize disease. There is no longer the complaint of the sick person, no longer anything to touch or to smell or to listen to. Images make disease much more comfortable for the physician; modern diagnostic images give the objectivity that we so prize in our model of science. The placebo brings us back to the patient, and it reminds me, at least, that one of the most important functions of the physician in the age of imaging triumphs is to act as the interpreter of the patient's complaints.

There are blind physicians, but are there deaf ones? The voice tells me so much. Physicians should look on images as giving them more time to listen than to talk with a person, but, at least in the hospitals where I have spent so much time, images isolate the patient from the physician.

I confess to the triumph I feel at looking at the image of what I had predicted from the patient's story would be there. It feels good to see the image, for my detective story is solved, and the problem is now "visualized." Listening to the same unraveling of the story, learning from patients the cause of their pain, does not give many of us that same thrill. That is really where the placebo is so important, because it reminds us that our job is to deal with complaints, not simply with disease. We need the quiet give and take of conversation. We need to sense the pragmatic approach of the law schools, which tells us that there are no permanent answers to the problems of people, though there may be permanent discoveries. The mystery of the placebo reminds me of the divergence of human knowledge rather than a forced convergence, which medical science and dogma seem to portend. It tells me that I should be more uncertain rather than more certain, that I should have faith in subjectivity as well as in objectivity, and that care—in that final phrase—is as important as cure.

Finally, placebo effects remind us that we physicians live in two worlds which sometimes seem to claim unequal loyalty. There is the world of science, in which drugs cure pneumonia and genetic triumphs change our lives. That is the written world, the world in which textbooks tell us of diseases. But we physicians live also in the instinctual world, the world of pain and suffering, of hope and joy, and that is the world of persons, the world we learn about from each other and from living—and suffering—with our patients, and so much more than from textbooks.

House officers, as indeed all practicing physicians, need to think more about the placebo, to use it as a gift for some patients, but most of all we should let the placebo remind us that we must be humble in our understanding and that our job is to take care of patients and not simply of diseases.

## References

Brody, H. *Placebos and the Philosophy of Medicine: Clinical, Conceptual and Ethical Issues* (Chicago: University of Chicago Press, 1980).

Jospe, M. *The Placebo Effect in Healing* (Lexington, Mass.: Lexington Books, 1978).

Ong, W. J. *Interfaces of the Word: Studies in the Evolution of Consciousness and Culture* (Ithaca, N.Y.: Cornell University Press, 1977).

# 14. *Lying*

**Ralph Crawshaw**

To tell the truth, physicians lie. But how can you believe they lie when you hear it from a physician, who must be a self-acknowledged liar? A pretty paradox this, which since ancient times has haunted the most trusted of professions made up of men and women who have always told most of the truth and sometimes more than the truth. To begin with, why would we physicians be so willing to swear a Hippocratic Oath if we were not aware of our wish to lie and conceal? But of course patients are aware in their hearts of our moral flaw, for who among them would want to hear, let alone bear, the truth, the whole unvarnished truth about their human condition. The doctor and the patient are joined in a tacit understanding that they should approach the truth, should nurture the truth, but need not worship the truth to the exclusion of the patient's well-being. As I say, what a pretty paradox, perplexing physicians as their lying extends through patients' lives, all the way from birth to death, from the profession's distant past into the foreseeable future.

But the tale to spin is not about a passel of well-paid liars pandering to the hypochondriacal whims of the public nor of a coterie of corrupt priests of science building a comfortable niche for themselves in a hood-winked society. What we are about is an attempt at understanding both sides of lying. One side is an intentionally misleading act or statement. The other side is truth saying, intentional, full disclosure in word and deed. By understanding them together we may better develop that essential to healing, trust, for without trust no therapy prospers. Only by understanding the care and nurturance of truth will our journey through the dark side of the doctor/patient relationship become worthwhile.

Henry Thoreau observed that it takes two to speak the truth, one to speak and another to hear, which could mean that patients lie as well as doctors.[1] Physicians, particularly psychiatrists, are keenly aware how patients as well as doctors lie, for it is a truism of psychotherapy that this week's interpretation (truth) is next week's resistance (lie). This phenomenon of converting a truth into a lie, one of the wonders of transference, works for both the patient and the doctor. Take, for example, the specialist who concluded the diagnostic workup of a young man with carcinoma of the rectum by answering the patient's question of how much longer he had to live with "Not long enough for us to ever become friends," a "truth" intended to maliciously mislead with confounding rejection. Experience teaches how easily both patient and doctor can become enemies of trust.

To make absolutely clear how few wish to know the whole truth and nothing but the truth, simply imagine a remarkably sophisticated computer capable of predicting the time of your death. It would model your life by tracing out your life-style, calibrating your genes, measuring the accumulation of sclerotic plaques per square millimeter of your blood vessels' surface, judging the risks connected with the form, extent, and destination of your travels, determining the degree to which you are exposed to violence, including nuclear holocausts, and report that you will cease to exist at 4:21 A.M., October 21, 2044, or, perhaps, tomorrow afternoon. Would you jump at the chance to get a copy of that computer readout?

Some people, in a burst of overwhelming curiosity, would rush to discover their fate, some would hesitate, others, burdened with soul-freezing dread, would attack the machine and attempt to destroy it. What would you do? Though this question of the whole truth becomes uppermost in your mind it can take a different form in the mind of your physician. The caring physician considers, since he or she is simultaneously an analog for the computer and your ally, whether all should be forced to know the truth. Should the computer readout be mandatory reading for you or should you know what you want to know and that is that?

It doesn't take our highly imaginary computer to put our common wish to be lied to into personal perspective. There is a high probability that each of us someday will be a patient, stretched out in a hospital bed, and a caring physician will enter our room, knowing that she can offer some comfort but no hope. Her question will be how much of the truth do you want to know and how do you want to go about hearing it. As the wise man says, it takes two to tell the truth, and we are back to our paradox that the most trusting of professions is sometimes trusted not to tell the truth.

## Bestiary of Lies

Agreeing that the quest for the holy grail of medical truth has more directions than a compass has points, we can, with a measure of humility, look closer at medical lying, its forms and processes. The taxonomy is daunting, for there are colored lies, white, yellow, and black, anatomical lies, barefaced and tall. There are protective lies, malicious lies, habitual lies, unconscious lies, fibs, perjury, deceits, exaggerations, evasions, excuses, myths, fictions, falsehoods, self-deceptions, quibbles, omissions, as well as ignorant, expected, institutional, scientific, and statistical lies, to name but a few. They are all intended to mislead and in their entirety make a veritable zoo of corrupt practices.

The best available classification of lying can be found in Sissela Bok's book on the subject.[2] She starts with white lies and moves through excuses to lies in crisis, lying to liars and enemies, lying for the public good, protective and paternalistic lies to the lies of science and medicine, all of which make a start at an inclusive outline of the possibilities for lying in our culture. However, for our purposes we do best to focus on purposeful misleading by physicians and how they may act as enemies of trust.

Given the size of our zoo of lies we cannot expect to make a complete survey of all the animals—neither time nor inclination permits such a scholarly approach. However, we can select a few beasts for close examination. I propose we look at white lies (rabbits), institutional lies (wildebeests), and self-deception (hyenas). Knowing these three inhabitants of our bestiary of prevarication will not make experts of us but should provide a workable cross section of our zoo and for the curious social naturalist open a way to identify other creatures when encountered in their native habitat.

## Physician White Lies

A white lie is one that is considered by the liar as trivial and harmless, much as those cute, long-eared, burrowing creatures, the rabbits, are considered as incidental to the great scheme of things. "So nice to see you," murmurs a harried physician to a patient, or "What a beautiful baby," the pediatrician says to an anxious mother—lubrication to smooth the way for an involved and difficult encounter, the doctor/patient relationship. Who ever heard of anyone hurt by a rabbit?

Take, for example, the white lie to the sick and weary filling a waiting room, announced albeit by the physician's surrogate, the receptionist, "Sorry, the doctor will be a little late as he is delayed by an emergency at the hospital." Occasionally this may be true but too often it is a white lie to cover the physician's dallying at lunch or a quick trip to the local marina to check the battery of his cabin cruiser.

My authority in judging this rabbit as a rabbit rests on the public's report. As president of the local medical society a few years back I let it be known through the media that I would be available Monday afternoons at society headquarters to hear the public's complaints, praise, and questions of the medical profession. All they had to do was call and make an appointment and I would listen. The public stopped by in numbers and over 50 percent of the complaints were of doctors wasting patients' time. There were, and presumably are, too many times that physicians were late to attribute it to emergencies. There were just not that many emergencies though there may be that many rabbits.

One man did not leave it at complaining to me. He wrote his physician, pointing out that the three hours he lost in the waiting room became money out of his pocket and he enclosed a bill for $45.00 to cover his lost time. The doctor, with the playful arrogance sometimes attributed to all the medical profession, wrote across the patient's bill that he had indeed wasted the patient's time but the patient was going to have a hard time collecting anything. The doctor was wrong, because the patient took the bill with the doctor's acknowledged lapse to small claims court and collected.

The prospect of all the patients in the nation collecting on such a prolific hutch of white liars is daunting to the imagination and should be frightening to the profession, yet this is but a minor incident compared to what medical answering-service operators, who live day-in, night-out with physician white lies, have to say. They report the prevalence of white lies to be too high for comfort.

Here are some examples of this cute beast gamboling innocently across the medical landscape: the doctor who asks the operator to page him at a certain time so he can get out of a meeting at a medical society or church. The doctor who refuses a call and tells the operator, "Just tell them you cannot find me." The doctor who has been paged many times by several operators and calls in to say that their inability to reach him must be due to operator error (however, when the operator requests a test call, the pager works fine). A doctor's wife who says he is out of town and she does not know who is on call. His associates insist the information is incorrect. Upon calling back to the residence the doctor answers the phone and takes the call. (How clear it is how lies can proliferate within families.)

At this point I feel a little uneasy, like a magician who, having succeeded in pulling a rabbit from a hat, goes on pulling more and more, unable to stop though he has the stage alive with bunnies. By simply moving to a different medical area and quizzing others—nurses, hospital administrators, emergency medical technicians, nursing home operators—how many physician white lies would appear and how many would we admit to patients? In fact, there are those physicians who believe white lies are good for patients and give therapeutic reasons for deception. The process is dignified with a name, placebo, translated from the Latin, "I please," and placebos are the March hares of medical white lies.

Placebos are medications not intended to have any therapeutic value beyond deceiving a patient into believing he or she is being helped. Placebos are the official, established, fully licensed white lies of the medical profession.

Dr. Howard Spiro has dealt with the question in detail, citing his own experience as a gastroenterologist and estimating that placebos have relieved the pain of peptic ulcer in approximately 60 percent of the cases.[3] He recommends the use of placebos if the physician keeps in mind that they "delude [physicians] into thinking their patient has no significant organic disease because the placebo relieves the patient's pain; find the placebo a first step to more major deceit or diagnostic ennui; or mistakenly believe that the placebo response indicates that the complaint is feigned," a sizable list of warnings to add to the label of this therapeutic dose even when it fails to include the dangers of introducing a foreign substance into a sick person's metabolism as well as a foreign concept into his or her psyche.

On the positive side, Dr. Spiro suggests that the placebo acts as a symbol signifying that someone cares and is doing something positive for the patient. This questionable icon at best is simply pleasing, at worst lying about possibilities for a relationship when there is no need to worry. If talking with patients helps, and it does for a number of reasons, it is enough to take the time to listen and talk, rather than surmise and escort the patient out the door with a promissory symbol of what may happen.

Not that the physician is alone in suggesting placebos. Again the patient is prone to use the questionable credibility of symbols when seeking a cure. A patient I saw insisted that she could not sleep without phenobarbital. Our sessions revolved around the wonders of that drug in taking her to an oblivion beyond insomnia and the suffering of her daily life. For me it was a placebo devoid of the ability of relieving her condition while keeping her depressed and dependent on magic. What she needed was help in overcoming her lowered self-esteem by constructively facing her reality, not fleeing from it. We were at loggerheads, with her demanding and me denying. Finally, I succumbed to her pleas and wrote her a prescription for one phenobarbital capsule with the instructions that it was to be used only when necessary and she was fully accountable to me for that necessity if she wished a refill. The psychotherapy prospered as she explored her fears, and she knew that if things got too bad she could resort to the magic pill. I altered the original condition and renewed the prescription about every six months not because she ever took it but because she carried the capsule in her change purse where it wore out in the rough and tumble of coins and keys. If the lady wished to lie to herself I was not going to zealously preach her out of her beliefs; however, neither was I interested in complicating her psychic or physiological defenses. She had enough troubles without adding my ignorance to them. We talked about her troubles in and out of the relationship without benefit of iatrogenic symbolizing.

What do these little white lies of medical practice cost? It is a little like asking what harm rabbits do. Harmless Easter bunnies hopping around a springtime pasture cannot be of much concern, unless you own the pasture and the prevalence of rabbits is enough to preclude other species. But in our profligate country the price of white lies may not be seen as exorbitant since the complaint is seldom raised to any significant degree. When we look just at prescribed drugs and not surgical or manipulative procedures or over-the-counter drugs, it is estimated that between 35 and 45 percent of all prescriptions are for substances that are incapable of having an effect on the condition for which they are prescribed, and at a sizable cost.[4] Thirty-five percent, the lower estimate, of the $28.75 billion spent in 1982 for prescription drugs yields a dollar cost of ten billion for but a portion of one form of medical lying.[5] Some rabbit patch that.

Should there be immediate concern about the white lies of doctors? Ask a nurse, receptionist, or answering-service operator about the plague of mistruths that disrupt communication about patient care and erode medical teamwork. Only an experienced concern which denies the tacit complicity of indifference will contain the pernicious affliction of these "harmless" creatures.

## Physicians' Institutional Lies

Few realize, including physicians, how seldom medical cultures encourage candor when dealing with the dying patient. Informing a patient suffering from a fatal disease of the diagnosis is difficult for both the patient and the doctor, so difficult that many believe it should be avoided. In fact, some medical schools and teachers instruct physicians in deceiving patients, which brings us to the institutional lie, another inhabitant of our zoo of prevarication. The institutional lie is a beast which moves in herds with accountability only to its fellow wanderers; that is, it goes where the herd goes and does what the herd does for the simple reason that "everyone does it." It is not lack of brains but "mass think" that makes the "dumb ox." Without the herd the ox knows not what to do but eat and work.

Rather than choose a local species of herd animal to exemplify the phenomenon of mass hypocrisy the universal nature of such deceptions is best seen at a distance and as foreign. Wildebeest, for example, live in large herds upon the African veldt close to water holes and when disturbed they dash away for a short distance, wheel around to confront what has frightened them with a toss of the head and a wild prance, and conclude with a meaningless buck and resumption of grazing.

The largest medical culture on earth in the largest country on earth, the Soviet Union, may be just such a herd and veldt where the institutional lie can flourish "because everyone does it." The Soviet medical culture by mandate denies knowledge of a fatal diagnosis for any patient. But the practice is common in other countries and is only unusual in the frank avowal of Soviet doctors of what in other countries such as Japan passes as simple custom, the instinct of the wildebeest.

A clinical example, from the experience of Dr. James Muller, a Harvard cardiologist, illustrates both the disruptive power of candor as well as the magnitude of expected medical deception in the name of patients' well-being.[6] In the course of collaborative cardiological research in Moscow, Dr. Muller was working on a small cardiac ward where a patient suddenly suffered a cardiac arrest. With immediate resuscitation Dr. Muller saved the sixty-three-year-old engineer but was called away from the scene before he could follow up with the patient. Later he returned and the convalescing patient asked him if his heart had actually stopped. The way he put it was, "Was I dead?" Dr. Muller was amazed that the patient had not been told about his condition and of the steps taken to save his life. He explained, "No, you were not dead. Your heart stopped beating briefly during the first hours of the attack, but we were able to supply blood to your brain by pumping on your chest." He then went on to explain in detail what had happened only to have the patient hug and kiss him on the cheeks in gratitude for his help. Dr. Muller was unaware that the encounter had been reported in detail to the director of the hospital, who called him into the office the next day and said, "Jim, in the Soviet Union we do not generally tell patients when a cardiac arrest has occurred. We feel such knowledge is often harmful to the patient's psychology, and in rare cases may lead to reflex cardiac arrest." There was no confusion in Dr. Muller's mind about what he should tell or not tell the next Soviet patient he might treat for severe cardiac disease.

My personal experience has been to have the head of Public Health in Leningrad, a creditable source, assure me that a Soviet physician never acknowledges a fatal diagnosis to a patient. At times he or she may confide the deadly prognosis to the family but always on the condition that the patient not be informed. Dying is not a shared experience in that country since everyone in Soviet hospitals has an "optimistic" diagnosis.

Such deception is part of the regular training of Soviet physicians. Their ethical training falls under the rubric of deontology, which is the philosophical study of duty where ethics is the study of choice. The outstanding Soviet academician and research physician N. W. Blokhin has written at length on the need to conceal unfavorable prognoses, emphasizing that "informing a patient in the last stages of a disease about the impossibility of aiding him is the equivalent of a death sentence and cannot be justified." [7]

This kind of medical lying is not as obvious as the white lie because it is hidden in the regular behavior of the herd which recognizes the lie as a universal good rather than an individual evil. The fear of patient and doctor together, largely unconscious, is institutionalized into a mutual denial as they shrink from the dreadful news that life is ending. Much the easier option is to play on the survival instinct of the patient with the unfounded hope that "surely something can be done." There is no placebo, pleasure, or pleasing for the judge who renders this verdict. By the very nature of physicians' training we are placed at odds with a fatal prognosis. Only as the physician is prepared to share courage with the patient can such news be conveyed honestly and compassionately. The truth of our mortality is there whether or not it is denied, and the essential question is, Do we have the strength to recognize it?

## Self-Deception: Physicians' Lies to Themselves

Undoubtedly the most difficult lies physicians have to deal with are the unconscious distortions of reality which we manufacture to make our lives seem, though not actually become, more tolerable. In childhood we all lie, the peak being between the ages of five and six, and boys seem more profligate with the truth than girls. We lie as children for a number of reasons ranging from simple playful imagination ("I killed a monster from outer space last night") to vanity ("My father has the best job in town") to fear ("I did not do it, Johnny did"). As we mature in the natural order of things we attempt to put lies behind us. It is part of the training a happy family imparts to its children. Yet the pattern of lying once established does not go away but retreats into a deeper part of our mind to wait and pounce on the truth when we least expect it, even into professional life.

In our bestiary these lies of self-deception are more than rabbits. They are hyenas, stinking, sculking scavengers, active day or night, in packs or alone, omnivorous to the point of devouring their own young, yet an integral part of the world. Because hyenas are retiring and characteristically flee at the least confrontation, like the unconscious lies of physicians they are difficult to observe and understand.

In fact, physicians' unconscious lies are so elusive I must cite a personal example. Late one night while on duty during my psychiatric training I was awakened by a telephone call from a duty nurse who exclaimed that one of the patients in the hospital had just been discovered in a suicide attempt. The nurse was distraught as she recounted how the patient had gone to the toilet, strung a belt around her neck and over a shower stall, and hanged herself only to be discovered by an alert aide. Would I come quickly, as the patient was unconscious? I listened, asked if the patient was breathing, ascertained that she was, and then explained to the nurse that since she was not my patient seeing an unfamiliar doctor would only disturb her more once she regained consciousness. With that I hung up, turned over, and started to go back to sleep. It took a full thirty seconds for me to recognize that my instantaneous, intellectual explanation why the patient was not my problem was a bare-faced lie. As I pulled on my trousers I called back, saying I would be there pronto. Ever since then I have remained alert to the laughing hyena which exists within me.

Unconscious lies plague the practitioner because their very nature is so deeply entwined with the wish to seem complete, to have the proper answer at the minimum emotional cost. These lies live on the carrion of our ignorance, so often wrapped in empty medical language. One of the most common such lies is that given by the surgeon to the recovering patient, "We got it just in time." What a miraculous figure the surgeon appears to be in the eyes of the patient, a savior of science, omniscient and omnipotent; that is, until he or she is asked to define "just in time." Does his or her fancied knowledge of the chronology of the patient's illness permit our omniscient surgeon equal glibness with the other side of his or her lie? Does he or she announce to the patient with equal certainty "We just missed getting it out in time"? I doubt it, since it is no longer a preening lie which feeds the surgeon's unconscious need for omnipotence. We can safely assume the latter lie will never be voiced at the patient's bedside.

But the most common form of this unconscious juggling of the truth occurs in assuring physicians they "know" because they have made a diagnosis. During the early part of this century Sir William Osler spent a good part of his professional life attacking the general diagnosis of "typhoid fever," a diagnosis which had replaced "ague" only to be abused in his day the way the diagnoses "virus," "allergy," and "stress" are abused today. Patients' vague symptoms are tidily wrapped up in deceitful packages to reassure physicians that they know when they do not know. It is a strange process in which the unconscious lie "a lot of that is going around these days" is not abandoned until a treatment is found for the specific disease which until then had been "going around a lot" as a lying cliché.

The wish to be seen as knowing is so strong among physicians that they often shrink from their ignorance, relying on the fact that the vast majority of illnesses which bring patients to them are self-limiting. Listening, as a psychiatrist, to a gastroenterologist decry family practitioners for treating gastric ulcers when they should refer the patients to him, the specialist, does little to increase my trust in the man. The distrust becomes intense when he proclaims he knows that 40 percent of these ulcers are caused by "stress" and he is the one best equipped to treat "stress" with antidepressants. His solipsistic belief does more than stimulate any rivalry I may have in garnering a full practice; it exposes to my view, if not his, the unconscious lie that he believes he knows.

The great problem with the physician's unconscious lie is how easily it is reinforced by an intellectual knowledge of the symptoms coupled with an immense and growing armamentarium of symptom-relieving drugs. These anodynes should never be denigrated because sometimes they are a blessing. However, these seductive drugs should always be viewed with a jaundiced eye as potential sources of dependency and interpersonal avoidance so much so that there is a need for a latter-day Homer to proclaim that one and all should beware of physicians bearing drugs.

In my practice the lie is uncovered when patients come asking, "Please, no drugs. I have been all through the antidepressant and co-deine routines from too many doctors. I want to know why I am shaky and cry so much." The patient seeks a truth which lies beyond physi-ology and pharmacology in an area where no physician "knows." Nor does the patient wish to learn my jargon of "identification," "counter transference," and "neurosis," ways in which I might scavenge off the patient's canker of symptoms. To help I must acknowledge that I do not know the source of the tears and tremors but will share in searching for their true cause—a process of truth thoughtful physicians learn through grim experience. I know because I have a hyena within me always ready to explain why I should not be intimately involved in the patient's search for health.

## Conclusion

What to make of physicians' lying? It is an acknowledged, perhaps nec-essary, ingredient of the practice of medicine. Yet it comes with a fearful price, for whether a white lie, an institutional lie, or self-deception, the alteration of the truth will in the long run lessen the effectiveness of the physician and will consequently hurt the patient.

Simple as it may seem, no treatment prospers without trust. Treat-ment can exist without trust but only to the degree that it is mechanical and thus fails to reinforce the complete healing process which calls for the patient's mind to have peace as well as his or her body to have strength. When a patient loses confidence and trust in a physician there is a dread-ful and destructive force set loose which finds expression in more than malpractice suits. Too often the loss is expressed as the patient's own loss of self-confidence. There is a dreadful loneliness which goes with disillusionment in those we love and depend upon, and ultimately we hold ourselves responsible—"I shall never trust again." Such disillu-sionment is corrosive to all that is healthy in a person or a people.

It is easy to deplore the times, claiming medical lying is an evil on the increase. Certainly the plethora of malpractice suits which plague to-day's medical profession is evidence that trust is suffering in the practice of medicine. The public attitude polls add to this conclusion by showing that in 1966, 72 percent of those asked had a great deal of confidence "in those who were running the medical care" while in 1981 this figure had dropped to 37 percent.[8] But it is not enough to cry havoc.

Though finding the cause of this loss of trust is more unyielding than simply decrying it, the cause can be uncovered. What it takes is a close and continuing appraisal of belief systems of physicians, patients, and the society. All must be honest about our dishonesty. This is the beginning premise to be clearly stated over and over.

Despite our animalness we need not despair. With all the faults and weaknesses which are so clearly part of present-day medical practice physicians can still be looked to as leaders in supporting the centrality of honesty, first, because their strength has grown through a science which honestly examines facts; second, because they have a traditional alliance and vast experience with the human condition; and third and most important, because physicians know no matter how difficult it may be that they serve their patients best by serving honestly.

The elemental reason why truth telling is indispensable for the physician is that for care to flourish there must be that special form of love called trust. Lies are poison to love and in large enough doses kill. The search for truth is eternal. Together in a bond of trust, patient and doctor have made much progress seeking that truth. We are healthier than ever before. Despite the complications of a vast technology and a complex delivery system, the human spirit can be expected to grow, fulfilling our complete capacity as human beings. So it is I share my true belief.

## Notes

1. Henry David Thoreau, *A Week on the Concord and Merrimack Rivers.*

2. Sissela Bok, *Lying* (New York: Pantheon Books, 1978).

3. H. Spiro, "Placebos, Patients and Physicians," *Pharos* 5, no. 47 (Spring 1984): 2–7.

4. Sissela Bok, "The Ethics of Giving Placebos," in *Ethics in Medicine,* ed. S. Reiser, A. Curran, and A. Dyck (Cambridge, Mass.: MIT Press, 1977), 251.

5. U.S. Bureau of the Census, *Statistical Abstract of the United States* (Washington, D.C.: U.S. Government Printing Office, 1984).

6. J. Muller, "Experiment in Moscow," *Notre Dame Magazine* 6, no. 4 (October 1977): 10–20.

7. N. W. Blokhin, "Deontology in Oncology," in *The Physician's Practical Library— Malignant Neoplasms* (Moscow: Medisina, 1977).

8. S. Lipset and W. Scheider, *The Confidence Gap* (New York: The Free Press, 1983), 48.

# Part IV.
*The Future for Physicianhood*

# 15. *The Future of Medical Practice*

Arnold S. Relman

The conditions of medical practice today differ substantially from those of the early 1900s and I believe it is important that physicians and non-physicians alike recognize that. I regard this historical perspective as essential to an understanding of why medical practice is being transformed by new forces.

The modern professional status of medicine in this country developed during the latter half of the last century and took final shape with the completion of the educational and licensing reforms that had been stimulated by the Flexner Report and spearheaded by the American Medical Association (AMA). By the early decades of this century, medicine was firmly established as the dominant and generally accepted health profession and it had the following characteristics: first, it was firmly rooted in the natural sciences, particularly biology and chemistry; second, it aspired to be rational and yet pragmatic, dependent on experience and the evidence; third, it was officially sanctioned and licensed by the state, but it was also largely self-regulated, self-credentialed, and self-disciplined.

(That, in essence, is the operating definition of a profession.) Most important of all for the purposes of this discussion, the practice of medicine was based on a special relationship between doctor and patient which is only briefly and inadequately described in the AMA's code of ethics and has had surprisingly little written attention from any sector of organized medicine.

The essential features of that special relationship are, first of all, that except in emergencies a physician is free to choose whom he or she will serve. But once he or she accepts responsibility to serve a patient, the physician is obligated to act as the trustee for the patient's interest and, whenever possible, with the patient's informed consent. In serving as the patient's trustee, the physician is expected to apply generally accepted professional standards of care, always for the patient's benefit. The patient's interest takes precedence over all other considerations—certainly over any financial or other personal interests of the physician. The latest edition of the *Opinions and Reports* (1981) of the Judicial Council of the AMA is very firm and explicit on this last point. It says, "Under no circumstances may the physician place his own financial interest above the welfare of his patient. The prime objective of the medical profession is to render service to humanity. Reward or financial gain is a subordinate consideration." You will note that the council does not say that financial gain is not any consideration. It merely says that such consideration should be subordinate to the patient's interests.

While the AMA's ethical code has never specified what form the physician's compensation should take, the assumption has always been, at least until recently, that the predominant mode would be fee-for-service. In accord with that assumption, the council's *Opinions and Reports* have over the years devoted much attention to the subject of fees and fee splitting.

Another important assumption in the early days was that patients would pay for their medical care *to the extent that they could afford it.* This necessitated that fees be reasonable and commensurate with the patient's ability to pay. Indeed, most editions of the *Opinions and Reports* until recently contained a statement that said, ". . . ability to pay should be considered in reducing fees; excessive fees are unethical."

We should recognize, however, that the fee-for-service arrangement, even when softened by charity, has always had an obvious and inherent conflict of interest for the physician. In economic terms, fee-for-service physicians are suppliers who are able to determine the demand for their own services. By virtue of their special knowledge, the authority vested in them by the state, and the trusting consent of their patients, fee-for-service physicians make the decisions to use the medical services that they themselves provide, and for which they will be paid on a piecework basis. It is a situation with a built-in potential for abuse, and the possibilities have not been overlooked by some of the sharpest critics of our society.

George Bernard Shaw, for example, wrote a devastating satire of private fee-for-service practice in the "Preface on Doctors" which accompanies his play *The Doctor's Dilemma*. He begins his preface this way:

> It is not the fault of our doctors that the medical service of the community, as at present provided for, is a murderous absurdity. That any sane nation, having observed that you could provide for the supply of bread by giving bakers a pecuniary interest in baking for you, should go on to give a surgeon a pecuniary interest in cutting off your leg, is enough to make one despair of political humanity. But that is precisely what we have done. And the more appalling the mutilation, the more the mutilator is paid. Scandalized voices murmur that . . . operations are necessary. They may be. It may also be necessary to hang a man or pull down a house. But we take good care not to make the hangman and the housebreaker the judges of that. If we did, no man's neck would be safe and no man's house stable . . .

Shaw wrote that in 1911. Despite his misgivings, private fee-for-service practice survived in the United Kingdom for another thirty-five years before it was largely replaced by the National Health Service. In this country the private fee-for-service has been more durable and more widely accepted. Until the past decade or two, it enjoyed the general confidence and support of the American public. There are many reasons for this. First of all, the behavior of most doctors was influenced by the ethical code of organized medicine, which clearly said that the whole system was based on the doctor's commitment to the patient's interests— the patient's interests were primary. Not only that, it was unethical for the doctor to do anything unnecessary. Of course, the chance of a physician doing anything unnecessary wasn't very great in the days when there weren't things for a physician to do beyond examining, counseling, and comforting.

Except for a relatively few surgical specialists, most doctors, most of the time, had only their time and advice to offer. Until forty or fifty years ago, the great majority of doctors in practice in this country were primary care givers who had only a modest and inexpensive array of procedures and remedies. When specialists were used, the referral usually came from the primary care physician, so self-referral by specialists was not a problem. The major ethical concern in those day was fee splitting between referring physician and specialist. But there weren't that many specialists around, and most medical care represented an ongoing personal commitment by a primary care physician. Doctors usually had to live with the consequences of their medical decisions, as patients did, because doctors and patients knew one another and doctors acted with a sense of personal responsibility that usually restrained any tendency to promote their own financial interests.

Furthermore, one of the most important protections against conflict of interest is disclosure, and disclosure is built into the solo practice, fee-for-service system. Patients consulting their physician know very well that if they choose to follow the doctor's advice to have some test or procedure carried out, the doctor expects to receive a fee for the service. If patients don't trust the integrity and judgment of their doctor, they can go to someone else, but there can be no deception about the nature of the arrangement because the physician's financial interest in the transaction is perfectly clear.

There was one final reason why the system worked pretty well. Until recently, doctors had more patients than they could handle. They really had no incentive to do more than was necessary for any patient because there were lots of patients out there and much work to do. As long as physicians were in relatively short supply, there was no pressure on them to offer their patients more than essential services.

Beginning just before World War II, the system of medical practice in this country began to change; after the war, new social and technological forces came into play that began to transform the profession and put new stresses on this simple satisfactory relationship between doctor and patient. One of the first and most important developments was the rise of specialism and an increase in the relative and absolute number of specialists. This in turn has led to the fragmentation of medical care and to less personal commitment by physicians to patients. We have changed from a system that had over 70 percent primary care physicians to one that now has nearly 70 percent specialists, and from a system in which patients rarely consulted a specialist without advice and referral from their general practitioner or family physician to one in which patients often refer themselves to specialists or are referred from one specialist to another, with *no* physician having responsibility for the coordination and continued follow-up of their total medical care.

Another major force that has changed the nature of the doctor-patient relationship is the explosive development of new medical technology. The increasing technological sophistication of medical practice and the enormous growth of its scientific information base are, of course, both a cause and a consequence of the growth of specialism. There are now a vastly increased number of things that doctors can do for patients—many more tests, many more diagnostic and therapeutic procedures, and many more identifiable, billable items to be reimbursed by the third-party payers. Doctors are no longer simply offering their time and counsel. Each new specialty offers an elaborate a la carte menu of specialized services, and each item on the menu has a price tag. Even generalists have an office full of equipment and procedures which can be deployed to supplement the traditional services of primary care.

An article in the business section of the *New York Times* of October 12, 1982, illustrates the point. It is headlined "New Tools in the M.D. Office" and it tells how "the health-care industry, seeking new profits in a potentially lucrative market, is moving diagnostic testing out of the medical laboratory and into the doctor's office." It then goes on to explain how "a new generation of diagnostic equipment designed for use in a doctor's office" is being developed and aggressively marketed with expectations of great profits for the companies manufacturing them. "Financial analysts say the new tests stand to increase the efficiency— and earnings—of doctors in private practice while improving patient care." The trouble with this glowing assessment by the "financial analysts" is that the medical evidence to support the widespread adoption of many of these new tests in routine office practice is lacking. The same can be said about many of the technologies now being so widely used in hospital practice—and I am referring not just to new gadgets and diagnostic tests but to the whole panoply of diagnostic and therapeutic procedures and special facilities that are applied in the practice of medicine.

I am not suggesting that physicians are inclined to use techniques known to be useless or unsafe. Not at all. The vast majority of physicians want to use only the technology that they believe will benefit their patients. The problem is that many tests and procedures simply haven't been adequately evaluated before they are used in practice, and there often isn't much reliable information about what is beneficial and what is not. New technology is being developed so rapidly and there is such pressure to apply it in practice, as the article in the business section of the *New York Times* makes clear, that evaluation of safety and efficacy has lagged far behind. It is frequently much easier and more attractive to develop and introduce a new test or procedure than to carry out rigorous, well-controlled clinical trials to determine whether it is safe and effective. Furthermore, even when a new medical technology has been adequately evaluated, it may be found to make only a small contribution to patient management, and the cost-benefit ratio may be dubious. Much medical decision making therefore concerns the use of tests or procedures that either have not been adequately evaluated or are of only marginal value, thus leaving physicians to rely on their own judgment in deciding whether or not to apply them in a particular clinical situation. As the technology revolution expands, so does the degree of uncertainty and the role of individual discretion in the practice of medicine. Judgment has always been important in medical practice, of course, but the personal consequences for patients and the economic stakes for physicians are now higher than ever before.

Finally, no description of the postwar changes in medical practice can ignore what many observers consider the most crucial development of all: namely, the rise of medical insurance and reimbursement by third parties. At the present time, around 85 percent of all patients in this country have some degree of third-party coverage, a system which up to now has reimbursed providers for their charges or for some agreed-upon schedule or fraction of their charges. Most third parties reimburse physicians on the basis of the so-called usual and customary rate (UCR) structure, a mechanism which gives incentives for the introduction of new specialists and new procedures.[1] With a fee scale that is primarily determined by the specialists themselves, the system rewards time spent doing procedures or tests far more generously than time spent examining, counseling, or managing patients. The third-party reimbursement system also had an important effect on the behavior of patients. They became claimants for medical care to which they felt entitled because the insurance premiums had been paid, and they had no personal interest in what things cost, since there were no out-of-pocket expenses. They therefore expected everything to be done that their doctor said needed to be done. Doctors, for their part, had no reason to be concerned about cost because they knew the insurance company would pay. And thus arose what the lawyers like to call the "moral hazard" of insurance: there was no professional or economic restraint on what was charged to insurance because of the view that it had already been paid for. But of course that kept driving up premiums and contributed to the rise in health care costs, which is such a major national concern today.

The most influential third-party payer is the federal government, which entered the scene in the mid 1960s. At that time the concept of health as every citizen's right was established and Medicare and Medicaid were passed into law. Expenditures in 1981 on these two programs alone amounted to more than $70 billion, or approximately 25 percent of the total cost of personal health care in that year. With this massive government commitment came a decline in the concept of charity and in the doctor's obligation to consider the patient's ability to pay in determining his or her fees. It is not surprising, therefore, that in the latest edition of the *Opinions and Reports* of the AMA's Judicial Council there no longer appears any statement about excessive fees or the physician's obligation to consider the patient's ability to pay.

Lest I appear to be lamenting the disappearance of the good old days of the two-class system, when doctors dispensed free care to the poor out of a sense of noblesse oblige, I want to make it clear that I consider Medicare and Medicaid to have been one of the major social advances of our time. You will note, however, that I use the past tense. New political policies in Washington and growing budgetary constraints in state and federal government are forcing cutbacks in these programs and moving us back toward the two-class system. Charity in the private sector may once again become the last resort for many of our elderly and indigent sick and disabled citizens. Nevertheless, the fact remains that most of our people do have some sort of health insurance, and this has powerfully contributed to the expansion of health care services in this country over the past several decades and to the changes that I have been describing in the medical profession.

Health insurance and third-party payment, coupled with increased specialism and the technology explosion, have been largely responsible for the rapid rise in health care expenditures and have created a new climate for medical practice in which there are virtually irresistible incentives for doctors to become entrepreneurial and profit seeking in their behavior. It has become so easy to exploit the money-making possibilities of medical practice that economic incentives now play a far more important role in determining the behavior of many physicians. By simply doing more procedures and tests, most doctors can do very well for themselves—far better than ever before   even as they try to do good for their patients. The technology explosion has provided the tools and insurance has removed the financial restraints on their use that doctor or patient might have felt in earlier times. As legions of new subspecialists graduate from training programs into this changed environment, they find it all too easy to take a fragmented, piecework approach to practice, leading inevitably to the excessive or inappropriate use of established procedures and the uncritical use of unproven new ones. In this climate, the conflict of interest that has always been inherent in the fee-for-service system takes on larger and more disturbing dimensions, and the practice of medicine in many instances now begins to resemble a business enterprise almost as much as a profession.

To illustrate what's happening in the practice of medicine today, I submit three items that have come across my desk in the past year or two. The first is a flyer sent to me by a physician in Missouri which he had received from a midwestern investment counseling company. It read, in part: "If you have been searching for a practical and prudent way to reduce taxes and increase your income, here is an excellent opportunity to do so. During the last three years, individuals and corporations earning in excess of $40,000 have purchased more than 1200 (blank) comput-erized ECG systems. A nationwide network of over 45 medical equip-ment distributors can place and service the system you purchase with other doctors in hospitals that actually use the equipment. The doctor or hospital using your equipment then pays you for each ECG they run, with a minimal monthly guarantee." The ad goes on to explain how the pur-chase and subsequent lease of this equipment provide a physician with depreciation, interest, and expense deductions which can lead to large tax savings.

Another example is a personalized ad that a physician in White Plains, New York received from the vice-president for marketing of a medical equipment corporation. It said: "Dear Dr.: You probably recognize the value treadmill exercise testing and Holter monitoring have in helping you deal more effectively with the epidemic incidence of coronary heart disease . . . but may have questions about the procedures and how they will fit into your setting. What better way to evaluate the role of either or both of these valuable procedures than to take advantage of this Spe-cial Offer. . . ." The ad then explains that the company will pay the doctor's travel and lodging expenses to attend a two-day professional educational seminar on exercise testing and Holter monitoring which is to be held in Maui, Hawaii. For those who purchase equipment, the company offers to pay all expenses for two for a week in a luxury hotel in Hawaii. They further offer to train the doctor's office staff and provide a sixty-day period to evaluate the procedure on a lease or rental basis. They also offer to reimburse the doctor the difference between billings and the rental during those sixty days. This kind of appeal evidently does not fall on deaf ears because the ad concludes this way: "We have assisted literally thousands of physicians to evaluate the role of these procedures in their setting. Let us send you referrals in your area."

These examples could be multiplied many times over in the private practice of medicine, but commercialism does not exist only among pri-vate practitioners, it is also to be found in the ivory tower. Many aca-demic clinical departments depend to an increasing extent on income earned from fee-for-service practice by full-time salaried faculty, and some of them are also being affected by the entrepreneurial spirit. Not long ago I received a letter about a manuscript being submitted to the *New England Journal of Medicine* from the cardiology section of a well-known academic department of medicine. There was nothing unusual about the letter, but the letterhead caught my eye. Under the university seal and the names of the members of the cardiology section, embla-zoned in large letters across the page, was the following advertising information: "Cardiovascular Consultations, Diagnostic Ultrasound,

Exercise Testing, Cardiac Rehabilitation, Intra-aortic Balloon Pumping, Cardiac Catheterization." The only thing lacking was a price list for the services being advertised.

In the last decade, new developments are compounding the problems I have been describing. First of all, not only have we had a change in the personnel mix, with relatively many more specialists and relatively fewer primary care physicians, but lately the total number of doctors has been increasing rapidly due to the expansion of medical schools. Over the past thirty years or so, there has been almost a doubling of the number of medical schools in this country, and more than a doubling of the number of medical school graduates. By the end of this decade, according to the Graduate Medical Education National Advisory Committee (GMENAC), which recently studied the employment situation very carefully, we will have about 536,000 physicians in this country. GMENAC estimates this number to be 70,000 more than the country will need. By the year 2000, the number of physicians will be 643,000, and GMENAC estimates that this will be 145,000 more than the country needs.[2] This rapidly expanding population of physicians is already increasing the competitive pressure on practitioners to generate more income by using marginal or new unproven procedures, tests, and technology. As the number of physicians continues to increase and as competition from outside the profession from nurse practitioners, chiropractors, and other kinds of health practitioners also expands, the pressure is bound to grow.

The second thing that has happened recently is a change in the government's attitude toward the practice of medicine. In 1975, in *Goldfarb v. Virginia State Bar*, the Supreme Court ruled that the professions are not exempt from the antitrust laws when it upheld a lower court's application of the Sherman Antitrust Act to the Virginia State Bar, which had attempted to establish and enforce a minimum fee schedule.[3] The Court said that this was price fixing in restraint of trade, implying that under the Sherman Act, the legal profession (as well as the medical profession) was a trade and that the government had a right to protect price competition. The Federal Trade Commission (FTC), which is the main regulatory body for enforcing the antitrust laws, has recently become especially interested in the medical profession and has already instituted several actions against organized medicine, the most notable of which was a suit against the AMA to prevent it from prohibiting advertising by physicians. The AMA at the moment is lobbying for new legislation that would exempt professions from the regulatory authority of the FTC but not from the jurisdiction of the antitrust laws. The administration seems to be encouraging commercialism in the practice of medicine, believing that price competition will help to hold down medical costs. The AMA, while hoping to escape from regulation by the FTC, does not seem inclined to make an issue of commercialism.

In the meantime, there has been an increase in the use of commercial advertising by physicians. A particularly flamboyant example appeared in the *New York Times* of January 22, 1982. It was a full-page ad by a group of plastic surgeons in New York called the "Creative Surgical Group." The ad had a bold headline that proclaimed: "You *can* do something about the way you look," and it featured some pretty slick copy. Here are a few samples: "Breasts can and should be beautiful. They needn't sag or balloon. What God did not give all women, we can. You would be amazed what an incredible difference it can make in a woman's attitude about herself. . . . Now your nose. Don't live with it if you don't think it's terrific. Noses are changeable. . . ." The advantages of face-lifts, otoplasties, and hair transplants were also touted with equal enthusiasm. The ad then offered readers a booklet on "a thoughtful review of cosmetic surgery" for $1.00 and ended with the reassurance that "all surgery is performed by Board-Certified plastic surgeons."

In discussing advertising by physicians, it is important to distinguish between the crassly commercial advertising of the kind I have just shown and what might be called informational advertising. The latter would be exemplified by a detailed professional directory or by an announcement of the availability of medical services. Informational advertising in my opinion is perfectly consistent with the spirit of medical professionalism, but commercial advertising that seeks to promote the demand for services is not.[4]

The fourth recent development, and I think perhaps the most significant of all, is the rise of what I have chosen to call the "new medical-industrial complex." The purpose of this article is not to dwell on this subject, which I have discussed in detail elsewhere.[5] But no consideration of the new commercial spirit in medicine can ignore this extraordinary phenomenon. Over the past ten or fifteen years we have seen the rise of a new kind of health care industry. These are businesses, usually large investor-owned corporations, that own or manage hospitals, nursing homes, clinics and emergency rooms, HMOs, diagnostic laboratories, dialysis centers, and a large variety of services and facilities that were formerly provided by private physicians. It is a huge and rapidly growing industry. It virtually began from scratch in the decade of the sixties and now accounts for roughly 15 to 20 percent of the personal health care delivery system in this country, with a gross income of probably more than $40 billion a year. This estimate does not include the pharmaceutical industry and the manufacturers of laboratory and hospital supplies and equipment.

The investor-owned hospital industry, which is one of the largest segments of the new medical-industrial complex, is consolidating into a few very large corporations that are gobbling up all the little fellows. There are now about five giant hospital corporations which control almost two-thirds of the investor-owned hospital market, which comprises about one thousand general hospitals in this country today. Some of these companies have sales of over two or three billion dollars a year. They market their hospital services just the way any profit-making company would be expected to and they're encouraging doctors to use their services.

Some of these companies put ads in the medical journals which in effect say to young doctors: "Where in the country would you like to practice? Would you like to practice in sunny Arizona, or in beautiful Florida or California? We'll take care of you." Young physicians send in their credentials and practice preferences and the companies place them in a hospital that they own or manage. They will set a new doctor up in practice. They arrange loans and guarantee the first year's income; they may offer a rent-free office for a year; they buy equipment if necessary. And all the physician has to do is agree to practice in their hospital.

Doctors are being wooed as customers of the investor-owned hospitals. But doctors all over the country are also investing in these companies and in many cases they are taking an active entrepreneurial role—founding and managing all kinds of health care businesses such as nursing homes, diagnostic laboratories, dialysis units, and so on. I don't know the exact extent to which this is happening—I doubt if anyone has accurate data—but I have the impression that it is very common for doctors to be investing in these profitable businesses. In doing so, physicians compound the conflict of interest that has always existed in fee-for-service medical practice, and they do it in a way that does not allow for disclosure. When physicians have financial interests in businesses that make profits by marketing health services to patients, the role of the physician as the trustee for the patient is called into question. How can the public be expected to have confidence in the profession, and how can the profession retain its own image of dedication to the public interest, when physicians become entrepreneurs in this way? It is a situation that challenges the character and spirit of the medical profession.

The key question is, Will medicine now become essentially a business, or will it remain a profession? Medical costs will have to be controlled; they are increasing to a degree that requires some sort of control. Will the medical profession do its share to help society solve the problems, or will it increasingly become part of the problem? Will we act as businessmen in a system that is becoming increasingly entrepreneurial, or will we choose to remain a profession, with all the obligations for self-regulation and protection of the public interest that this commitment implies? If we wish to remain a profession, we're going to have to deal with the problems I have been describing. This is not the place to discuss in detail what I think needs to be done, but I offer in brief outline seven suggestions for initiatives that would reassure the public and help restore the image of the medical profession as being responsive to the needs of the public and the interests of patients.

In the first place, I think we should address the medical personnel problem in a more positive way to deal with the impending problem of physician overproduction. We will need to look not only at the physicians we're producing in the United States, but at the thousands who are being educated in fourth-rate "offshore" medical schools and coming back into the American system through the back door.[6] Most of all, we will have to address the problem of the imbalance between primary care physicians and specialists. Regardless of what one thinks about the absolute number of physicians needed in the future, there is a clear consensus among the experts that something should be done to increase the proportion of primary care physicians and this will require concerted action by all those responsible for graduate medical education.

Second, organized medicine, together with the third-party payers, should change the relative value scale for medical fees. Physicians will need to deal with the problem caused by our present policy of rewarding procedures, tests, and technology far more generously than primary care. As long as the fees for procedures and specialized services are so much higher than those for personal services, there is little chance that primary care will be successfully encouraged or that we will reverse the trend toward commercialism and excessive use of fragmented a la carte medical services.

Third, organized medicine should be more active in controlling the quality of health care in this country. To restore public and governmental confidence in the ability of the profession to regulate itself, organized medicine will have to take more vigorous action against quacks and frauds and impaired physicians. It's going to have to police itself more effectively than it has ever done before.

Fourth, the medical profession should push for a national program of technology assessment.[7] I do not know whether such a program should be based in government or the private sector, but there is urgent need for a new mechanism of funding clinical trials to evaluate health care procedures, and organized medicine should do its part in supporting constructive efforts in this direction. New clinical trials and new data are needed, not simply pronouncements by committees based on inadequate available information. Physicians should be lobbying for new funding mechanisms to pay for the gathering of new data. Provided that practitioners have access to the new data and modify their practices in accordance with the new findings, such a program is bound not only to improve medical practice but to save large sums of money now being wasted on unnecessary, ineffective, or unsafe procedures. Technology assessment and the proper uses of such information in medical decision making should be given more attention in undergraduate medical education.

Fifth, we should support experiments with new forms of medical care organizations that give incentives to reduce unnecessary hospitalization and promote more efficient practice. Organized medicine should be more receptive to experiments like HMOs and primary care networks. All too often in the past, established professional groups have resisted such experiments, leading to the public impression that they were sometimes more concerned about their own economic interests than the public welfare.

Sixth, the medical profession should support improvement and rationalization of the hospital reimbursement system. We should support the prepayment approach and encourage the institution of cost-control incentives. But, as we move to a system of prospective payment, one that gives the hospital an economic incentive to be more efficient and less expensive in its management of patients, the incentives for physicians for the first time may be in direct opposition to the incentives for hospitals.[8] It may be in the doctor's economic interest to have more money spent on hospitalization, whereas with prospective payment, hospitals may benefit from spending less. Physicians will have to face up to that problem and deal with it responsibly—not simply by setting up diagnostic and treatment facilities in their offices that will compete with the hospitals.

Finally, but perhaps even more important than any of the other points, the medical profession should publicly and clearly separate itself from the health care industry. It should declare as an article of its ethical code that doctors should derive income in health care only from their professional services and not from any kind of entrepreneurial interest in the health care industry. In my view that would be the best way to reaffirm the credibility of the medical profession and demonstrate its entitlement to a continuation of the implicit social contract that exists between medicine and the public.

The public gives doctors special advantages and privileges in exchange for a commitment to put the public's interests ahead of any personal economic gain. Ipso facto, involvement of practicing physicians as investors or entrepreneurs in the "new medical-industrial complex" raises serious doubts about this commitment. Physicians should be fiduciaries or representatives for their patients in evaluating and selecting the services offered by the health care industry; they cannot ethically serve in that capacity if they also have financial interests in that industry.

A commitment to these seven initiatives would, in my opinion, be clear evidence that the medical profession wishes to meet its public responsibilities as a profession and that it does not regard itself as simply a highly skilled business or trade. These initiatives are not the only, or necessarily the best, ways to solve the problems I have outlined here, but I believe they are a good way to begin. If we cling to our present course, I am convinced that the independence and ethical base of our profession will be progressively eroded and the practice of medicine will continue to evolve into commerce. The marketplace will dominate, the Federal Trade Commission will become more active, and the medical profession will see more federal regulation. We may have trouble with the Federal Trade Commission in any event, whatever the medical profession does, but I believe that the problem can be worked out if the medical profession is seen to be acting in the public interest. Failing that, there may well be a progressive weakening of the fee-for-service system. Already almost 50 percent of all physicians are salaried; even excluding house officers, almost 40 percent of physicians work for a salary.[9] In the absence of any kind of professional self-regulation, that percentage will continue to grow. Doctors will more and more become employees. Doctors' unions, which already have forty or fifty thousand members, will become even more powerful. Doctors will ultimately function less as independent professionals and more as businessmen or employees in a commercial market. Paul Starr's prediction of the imminent decline of medical professional sovereignty may well come true.[10]

The choice between this course and continuation as responsible, independent professionals is in the hands of the profession, particularly the new physicians. Although the problems were generated by external social and economic forces and by inevitable technological changes, the predicament that I've described is basically an internal moral crisis. We have the means to solve our problems if we but choose to do so.

## Notes

1. Benson B. Roe, "The UCR Boondoggle: A Death Knell for Private Practice?" *New England Journal of Medicine* 305 (1981): 45–50.

2. U.S. Department of Health and Human Services, *Report of the Graduate Medical Education Advisory Committee,* September 1980.

3. *Goldfarb* v. *Virginia State Bar,* 421 U.S. 773 (1975).

4. Arnold S. Relman, "Professional Directories—But Not Commercial Advertising—As a Public Service," *New England Journal of Medicine* 299 (1978): 476–478.

5. Arnold S. Relman, "The New Medical-Industrial Complex," *New England Journal of Medicine* 303 (1980): 963–970.

6. Arnold S. Relman, "Americans Studying Abroad: We Need a New Policy," *New England Journal of Medicine* 299 (1978): 1012–1014.

7. Arnold S. Relman, "Assessment of Medical Practices: A Simple Proposal," *New England Journal of Medicine* 303 (1980): 153–154.

8. John K. Iglehart, "The New Era of Prospective Payment for Hospitals," *New England Journal of Medicine* 307 (1982): 1288–1292.

9. Henry S. Kahn and Peter Orris, "The Emerging Role of Salaried Physicians: An Organizational Proposal," *Journal of Public Health Policy* 3 (1982): 284–292.

10. Paul Starr, *The Social Transformation of American Medicine* (New York: Basic Books, 1982).

# 16. *Technology and the Eclipse of Individualism in Medicine*

Stanley J. Reiser

In little more than 150 years two revolutions that have changed the way doctors evaluate disease have taken place in medicine. The first has to do with the refinement of physical diagnosis and the second with the emergence of technological diagnostic techniques. These developments have created critical shifts in the doctor-patient relationship and in the physician's individualism.

The first diagnostic revolution occurred in the second decade of the nineteenth century. Until that time physicians practiced primarily at a physical distance from patients. Interdictions against manipulation of the body with hand or instrument stemmed from the association of such activities with the surgeon, then considered the inferior of the physician by dint of social class and erudition. Physicians evaluated illness principally through two techniques: learning the patient's experiences through questioning and listening, and visual inspection of the body.

This nonphysical and nontechnical approach to diagnosis was challenged successfully in 1816 by a French doctor, René Laennec. Puzzled by the illness of an obese young woman with heart trouble and finding traditional diagnostic methods unavailing, Laennec thought that he might possibly learn something by trying a long-standing but seldom used method of inquiry—listening to sounds made by the organs of the chest. To do so required placing an ear directly upon it. This Laennec, with modesty typical of this era, could not bring himself to do, citing the age and sex of the patient as deterrents. A thought then flashed through his mind: solid bodies augment sound. He seized a sheath of paper from the table adjoining the bed, rolled it into a tube, brought one end to his ear, and placed the other end on the patient's chest. The sounds that emerged convinced him that here might lie a treasure of valuable diagnostic signs that none before him had systematically attempted to mine. Using a tube similar to that first created from the paper but now made of wood and christened the stethoscope, he explored chest sounds for three years. What finally emerged was the treatise *De l'auscultation médiate.*[1] It convincingly argued that the physical evidence gleaned directly through the doctor's senses constituted data about illness superior to that gained from the experiences and sensations described by the patient. The book also caused the first widespread adoption of an instrument in diagnosis, the stethoscope.

These early days of physical diagnosis were heady ones for doctors. Now freed from the inhibitions directed against physical manipulation, they followed the lead of Laennec exploring with their senses, aided sometimes by simple instruments, all aspects of the body. With each major advance in exposing the body's organs to direct sensory observation, the prospects for physical diagnosis became all the more exciting. Reaction to the laryngoscope, introduced in 1855, was typical: "The man of experience," wrote a doctor, "has now only to *look* into the larynx, and he will *see* what is the form of the disease with which he has to deal."[2] Or, "May it not be said without exaggeration, that it has rendered the diagnosis of the diseases of the larynx more simple and more certain than the diagnosis of the diseases of any other internal organ? In fact the larynx has ceased to be an internal organ, in the sense of being hidden from view, for it has been brought within the range of vision."[3]

Exhilaration over the possibilities of physical examination was matched by growing dismissal and suspicion of older techniques of clinical evaluation, such as the evidence patients had to give. Doctors complained that when questioned patients were often too talkative or introduced irrelevant data, or that when anxious they might exaggerate symptoms, or that when shy or embarrassed about a condition they might withhold evidence. The intensity of symptoms could vary with personal idiosyncrasy or nationality. Not only patients but doctors damaged and altered historical evidence. By asking leading questions based on preconceptions formed of a case the doctor could change the reported character of subjective symptoms and make the patient's story conform to his view.[4] One clinician, whose dispensary relied almost entirely on physical examination, explained the situation plainly: "We may, after eliciting . . . [the patient's] history as 'sick at the stomach, headache, constipation,' and, the greatest of all symptoms, 'don't feel right,' find, by physical examination, some heart lesion, nephritis, or other serious disease."[5]

The second diagnostic revolution began as the nineteenth century drew to a close. While physicians were gaining skill in the use of their own senses to evaluate illness, instruments were being developed that made the exercise apparently unnecessary. The new technologies had the capacity themselves to sense evidence and, most critically, to transform it into the objective forms of pictorial, graphic, or numerical data. They were far more complex than the instruments such as the stethoscope that doctors used in the era of physical diagnosis. Many had their origins in the newly developing laboratories of physiology, biological chemistry, and bacteriology. The instruments stood for high science; they were its representatives at the bedside.

Typical of the graph-generating machines was the clinical polygraph, introduced in the 1880s by the British clinician James Mackenzie to depict irregular heart action. The apparatus particularly conveyed to patients the feeling of "science" at work, at once precise, mysterious, unknowable to all but those initiated into its ways: "Watch the drum as it revolves slowly," wrote an English doctor, "[watch] . . . the pens, like the sensitive antennae of some monstrous insect, trace their white lines on the smoky surface of the paper. Or, again, watch the doctor as he 'smokes' his paper over the burning camphor, like some priest of ancient cult performing a strange rite. What would not the 'worse end' of Harley Street have given for this 'business'?"[6]

This machine, and its more refined later models, drew enthusiastic reactions from heart specialists all over Europe and the United States. Many used the instrument believing that purchase of the hardware also brought the wisdom its inventor extracted from it, by linking the graphic recordings with a careful study of clinical symptoms at the bedside. Mackenzie denounced blind worship of machines in medicine. The polygraph, like other technologies, was for him means to illuminate patients' descriptions and the sensory findings of physicians. He thought of it mainly as a tool for research. "For routine practice," he wrote, "no instrument is necessary, and as soon as I had found out the knowledge it could convey, I set about discovering means by which the information could be obtained by the unaided senses."[7] Mackenzie's view was extreme for his time. Few saw as he did the limitations of the new technology. Few since have attempted as he did systematically to extract histori-cally or physically based clinical knowledge from technologic data.

Development of techniques of analysis applied in laboratories was equally significant in changing the diagnostic behavior of physicians. While machines like the polygraph were used by the expert at the bed-side, techniques of analyzing fluids and solid tissues did not require the presence of patients at the site of investigation, only parts of them con-veyed in vials and bottles to experts situated in laboratories. The new chemical and microscopical techniques produced a breed of medical specialists who seldom ventured to the bedside. They could conduct ex-aminations and dispense judgments at a distance from physician and pa-tient. The prototypic figure of this kind was the bacteriologist. In the 1880s medicine was turned topsy-turvy by convincing proofs that the world of microorganisms, known to exist for several centuries by scien-tists, was responsible for many of the major epidemic diseases afflicting people. These revelations converted the medical laboratory, which had been developed to advance basic understanding of biologic process, also into a place where diagnostic analyses of the problems of patients were conducted. Perhaps more than any other institution the laboratory sym-bolized to doctor and patient the arrival of science in medicine. Its elabo-rate analyses and findings, often dispensed in quantitative form, seemed dependable and sure.

With these developments diagnoses made basically from sensory ob-servations of doctors began to diminish. S. Weir Mitchell in his 1891 presidential address to the Congress of American Physicians and Sur-geons told his colleagues, "You know, alas! that we now use as many instruments as a mechanic."[8]

By the second decade of the twentieth century a distinction was wide-spread between those "modern" doctors drawing upon the laboratory for evidence and those "others" who continued to rely on physical data gained from bedside examination made themselves. At Harvard Medi-cal School this distinction was the basis for a virtual split of the faculty into two separate factions. It was the prevailing notion that machine-generated and laboratory evidence stood for exactness and precision—for science; that clinical evidence stood for diversity and vagueness—for empiricism. "The bacteriologist is tempted to form a mental picture of the day when the methods of bedside diagnosis . . . will be rendered superfluous; when the laboratory will supply a clear-cut diagnosis, cer-tainty in place of doubt," wrote Archibald Garrod.[9]

People clamored for access to new tests such as the Wassermann reac-tion for syphilis. Introduced in 1906, it became symbolic of the new power science had given to doctors. The Wassermann seemed infallibly to detect disease in the symptomatic and in the asymptomatic patient as well: a negative finding immediately calmed those obsessed with the idea that they had syphilis. Perhaps more than any other test it encouraged patients to seek laboratory aids to diagnosis, and doctors to use them.[10] To laymen as well as medical professionals, nontechnological methods seemed no longer sufficient to find disease: "As a means of gaining the confidence and retaining the control of our patients," wrote a doctor, "the laboratory diagnosis often places us in a position of such absolute certainty as to leave no doubt in the mind of the patient of its accuracy." [11]

Wanting to believe that through the use of technology medicine was emerging from an art to a science, physicians attributed levels of accuracy to the technology that it did not have. The numbers generated by the laboratory, like the linear waves produced by the polygraph, represented to them evidence that seemed detached in some way from human involvement. The machines, the chemical tests—all were embodiments of a pure science. Somehow, it appeared to doctors, no matter how instruments were constructed, maintained, or applied they would generate a uniform result which would be self-evident and unaffected by human judgment. One physician, speaking the feelings of many, called upon colleagues to substitute for "the immediate sense perceptions and personal judgments of the physician, methods carrying a capacity for numerical values and graphic record-methods, that is to say, which may be relied on to yield results unaffected by the personal bias or other defects of the individual observer." [12] Medicine had acquired an appetite to purge subjectivity from its ranks. Science, through medical instruments, seemed to provide a means to do away with clinical diversity and the error and controversy that accompanied it. Technological and chemical sensors would get things right. What doctors then as now remained generally unaware of was the large rate of error associated with machines and their users—15 to 20 percent on the average, as revealed by a 1975 study.[13] Results for prior decades were worse. Physicians continued to forget that behind every machine was a human mind.

Could the power to apply these instruments remain in the hands of individual doctors? Some thought yes, given will and training. William Osler urged physicians never to allow others to examine urine specimens for them.[14] Some argued that young doctors particularly, schooled in the ways of the laboratory, could apply the technology themselves or at least employ assistants working under their watchful eye. Only in this way could laboratory and bedside evidence be properly combined. Yet this linkage was not to develop: "Physicians do not supervise their own laboratory work sufficiently," complained a doctor in 1910. "They have the work done at a distance from home and thus lose, in a measure, the most important relationship between the laboratory findings and the clinical picture as manifested in the patient." [15]

The tide that produced the growing delegation of diagnostic judgments to technical consultants had several components. One was an improved communications network that allowed the rapid transmission of specimens and findings. Turn-of-the-century doctors used automobiles to get material to laboratories and the telephone to gain results. Even rural practitioners, using the train and the telegraph, now began to feel connected to medical science. They spoke of laboratories being almost as near to them as to physicians in the city. [16] Promise of even more spectacular gains in communicating medical evidence over distances emerged in 1905 from the laboratory of Willem Einthoven. He transmitted over wire electrocardiograms (he called them telecardiograms) of patients' hearts from his laboratory to the Leyden Hospital 1.5 kilometers away. Medical practice has yet to seize the advantage of such long-distance diagnostic possibilities. [17]

Improved communication made delegation easier. But other factors were more significant for the process. Many of the new diagnostic methods were too complicated or time-consuming for the average physician personally to use or oversee. Equipment was costly, and the skills needed to apply it could be maintained only by constant involvement with it and the test materials. [18] And perhaps most important, clinicians relied too much on technology to depend on themselves; what they needed were experts.

To become expert in medicine beginning in the early decades of the twentieth century meant becoming a specialist. Medical students increasingly viewed specialists as the main repository of accurate knowledge. Only specialists, schooled in a particular aspect of medicine, could hope to sort out the crowd of instruments and techniques waiting to be mastered. "So vast is the extent of knowledge to be gained of disease that no one man can hope to accomplish more than a small share during his lifetime. The old-time family practitioner has passed away and with him has passed individualism in medicine," wrote William Mayo in 1912. [19] By 1930 the growth of specialism among doctors had accelerated: then almost one of four limited practice to a particular medical subject. Today more than four doctors in five hold specialist credentials. While the attention of medicine has focused on the specialist activities of physicians, there has been a relative inattention to the effects of specialism within the growing community of allied health personnel and nurses.

At the beginning of the twentieth century about 345,000 people worked in health care, and about 1 out of 3 were physicians. Most of these others

who were not doctors were nurses. By 1940, the specialization of the
nonphysician work force was keeping pace with specialization among
doctors. Then some 27 new and recognized nonphysician occupations
existed, including physical therapy, dental hygiene, radiologic technology, and medical technology. By 1976, the health work force had grown
to about 5.1 million, and only 1 out of 13 in this group were physicians.
Moreover, the number of recognized specialties in the nonphysician
work force had now outpaced that within medicine. The allied health
occupations alone (which excludes nursing and nurse auxiliaries) contained 155 recognized specialties in 1976. Many specialists were created by technology, such as the specialist in blood bank technology, the
chemical technologist, the cytotechnologist, the emergency medical
technician, the environmental engineering assistant, the health physics
technician.[20]

The presence of so large a body of people assuming a growing responsibility for the application of technology in medicine warrants attention. Considerable evidence exists that variations in education and
conditions of work, in physical and psychological distance from the patient and treating physicians, and in understanding the influence of instrumental findings on the well-being of patients produces uneven rates
of competence among individuals in this group. How then to educate allied health specialists so that they understand the problems of responsibly using technology? What organizational structures are needed to
foster adequate interaction of allied health workers with each other, and
with physicians, to coordinate patient care? How does the intimate relation of these technically trained personnel to the technology they use
affect the exchange of clinical data with physicians, who often know
less about the technology than the technician but are responsible for
making clinical decisions? All difficult questions, but ones we must
answer.

When William Mayo spoke in 1912 of the passing of "individualism"
he defined one of the characteristic effects of technology on modern
medicine, expressed in the developments I have outlined. The techno-
logically induced waning of individual capacity to select and synthesize
evidence, to determine and justify action, is a central feature of medical
life in the twentieth century and a major problem. Can we cope with it?
I believe yes.

A crucial dimension of this problem is the matter of delegation. The
more we know about the causes and effects of illness the more tools we
develop to probe and treat it. As such tools proliferate fewer doctors
have first-hand knowledge of each particular one, and any given physician has to accept the judgments of more and more others in diagnosing
and prescribing for a patient. Outside the sphere of a particular spe-

cialization, which encompasses an ever more narrow domain with the passage of time, no physician is an authority. As these developments proceed unimpeded, physicians increasingly assume the role of middlemen, passing on to patients the authoritative views of experts. The principal medical judgment becomes less clinical—the personal obtaining and evaluation of evidence—and more managerial—the selection of consultants.

As a first step to resolving this dilemma, there is a need for medical students and house staff to develop an integrated view of the uses and purposes of technology. Currently, students encounter technology randomly, piecemeal, as the need arises in clerkships or residencies. They are not exposed to systematic consideration of such questions as, Why or how is one to assess a technology's effectiveness? How can one use technology without becoming dominated by it? How does one choose potential recipients of technology when resources are limited? How much should one spend on it and pay for it? How can one apply technology to improve the efficiency and coordination of patient care? How does one govern technology without stifling innovation or hampering patient care? A coordinated pedagogic approach to technology use is essential in medical education. To meet this need the National Center for Health Care Technology and other health agencies are sponsoring the development of teaching materials aimed at improving the physician's ability to apply technology effectively and humanely in patient care and helping to end the state of ignorance about technological medicine.

A second major resource to sustain independent judgment in medicine is a machine itself—the computer. Computers were introduced into clinical medicine at the beginning of the 1960s. At the time physicians felt stifled by the burden of growing mountains of facts they could neither sort well nor store adequately. Relatively little progress has been made since in adopting computers in practice. Clinicians who understand how computer programs are developed and how computers work can take advantage of their enormous potential to store, retrieve, and compare all kinds of medical evidence. Such an analytic instrument, applied by users aware of its failings and unthreatened by its powers, can greatly extend their capabilities to function as independent decision makers. Computer literacy, like general technologic literacy, should be an important goal of medical education.

A third response to the dilemma of dependency is finding a resource to apply alongside of technology in evaluating disease, one that uses human-centered skills, that gives physicians a sense of self-confidence and independence, that can be applied ubiquitously to probe illness, that is not endangered by obsolescence. The clinical interview is such a resource. The power to assess the needs of a patient seeking medical help, to formulate from the patient's experiences a diagnostic and prognostic view of what is wrong, to explain to the patient what should be done, and to monitor the results of subsequent intervention can be gained through knowledgeably conducted clinical interviews. One of the tragedies of twentieth-century medical education is that an intense focus on teaching technological skills has produced a relative neglect of available information about human communication and a failure to train physicians to apply words (and silences) as precisely and effectively in treating illness as they are taught to apply scalpels. Throughout this century social scientists, psychologists, and information and systems theorists have accumulated data about how communication works. In the same period reduction in the size and cost of videorecording equipment makes possible the taping and playback of interviews with patients. Now for the first time in the history of medicine we can get accurate documentation of what really happens in the clinical encounter. But few do.

Despite all that we know and have, clinical interviewing is usually taught in a random, unstructured way. Over the entire span of their medical education, most students in American medical schools are directly observed by instructors little more than once while conducting an interview.[21] Few schools provide structured, intensive courses in the interview process. Such courses as are offered are usually elective and taken by a minority of students. Yet the evidence provided by the skillfully conducted interview is invaluable in gauging the cogency or accuracy of technological procedures and data, the validity of which clinicians often cannot directly judge. The interview can generate significant data about the needs and problems of illness unobtainable through any technological mode of evaluation.

Finally, it is important to begin to examine what the emerging interdependence of people and machines in medicine foreshadows. Machines are complex entities which reflect human power and also weakness. We must recognize that we build ourselves into machines; that when we confront their powers we confront our own purposes, that when we accept their results we accept our own uncertainties. We must see that as machines become more numerous and ubiquitous in our daily lives we share more of our existence with them. Machines demand relationship. They do things to us just as we do things to them. Still, the powers we give machines that command and shape us diminish as we come to understand their effects on us and develop the capability to co-exist with them. Perhaps what frustrates us most is that total control of the machines we build eludes us. They seem like things but influence like people. In part, they possess capacities that are ours. But only in part. For what machines can never have are those qualities at the core of human civilization—a sense of the ethical, a kinship with suffering, a view of the past, a vision of the future.

## Notes

1. R. T. H. Laennec, *De l'auscultation médiate* (Paris: J. A. Brosson and J. S. Chaude, 1819).

2. A. Ruppaner, "The Practice of Laryngoscopy and Rhinoscopy," *New York Medical Journal* 6 (1867): 14.

3. G. Johnson, "Two Lectures on the Laryngoscope," *Lancet* 1 (1864): 604.

4. J. H. Musser, *A Practical Treatise on Medical Diagnosis for Students and Physicians* (Philadelphia: Lea Brothers, 1894), 30–32.

5. H. D. Marcus, "Thorough Physical Examination versus the Patient's Statement," *Medical Bulletin* 17 (1895): 401.

6. R. M. Wilson, *The Beloved Physician* (New York: Macmillan, 1927), 77.

7. J. Mackenzie, *The Future of Medicine* (London: H. Frowde, Hodder and Stoughton, 1919), 94–95.

8. S. W. Mitchell, "The History of Instrumental Precision in Medicine," *Boston Medical and Surgical Journal* 125 (1891): 311.

9. A. Garrod, "The Laboratory and the Ward," in *Contributions to Medical and Biological Research, Dedicated to Sir William Osler in Honour of His 70th Birthday, July 12, 1919, by His Pupils and Co-workers* (New York: Paul B. Hoeber, 1919), 63.

10. W. P. Lucas, "The Wassermann Reaction in Its Application to Medicine," *Boston Medical and Surgical Journal* 169 (1913): 116–117.

11. A. C. Kimberlin, "The Psychologic Value of a Correct Diagnosis," *Journal of the Indiana State Medical Association* 5 (1912): 271. See also G. Dock, "Laboratory and Clinical Examinations," *Journal of Laboratory and Clinical Medicine* 1 (1915): 23; and "Intensive Diagnostic Methods," *Boston Medical and Surgical Journal* 176 (1917): 510–511.

12. C. O. Hawthorne, *Studies in Clinical Medicine* (London: John Bale, Sons and Danielsson, Ltd., 1912), 164.

13. L. M. Koran, "The Reliability of Clinical Methods, Data and Judgments," *New England Journal of Medicine* 293 (1975): 700.

14. W. Osler, "Organization of the Clinical Laboratory," *British Medical Journal* 2 (1914): 335.

15. P. H. Ringer, "Abuse of the Clinical Laboratory from the Standpoint of the Laboratory-Worker," *Journal of the American Medical Association* 55 (1910): 530.

16. C. K. Beck, "The Rural Physician and the Diagnostic Laboratory," *Kentucky Medical Journal* 15 (1917): 384.

17. S. J. Reiser, *Medicine and the Reign of Technology* (New York: Cambridge University Press, 1978), 196–202.

18. T. W. Hastings, "Reciprocal Relations of the Clinic and the Laboratory in Medicine," *Journal of the American Medical Association* 61 (1913): 652.

19. W. J. Mayo, "Contributions of the Nineteenth Century to a Living Pathology," *Boston Medical and Surgical Journal* 167 (1912): 754.

20. National Commission on Allied Health Education, *The Future of Allied Health Education* (San Francisco: Jossey-Bass, 1980).

21. G. L. Engel, "Are Medical Schools Neglecting Clinical Skills?" *Journal of the American Medical Association* 236 (1976): 861–863.

# 17. *The Humanities and the Arts in Medical Education*

Roger J. Bulger

In April 1971 an interdisciplinary conference sponsored by the Society for Health and Human Values was held at Arden House in Harriman, New York to explore the desirability and implications of formal attempts to bring scholars and teachers of the humanities into the structure of medical education in a significant way. Philosophers, theologians, historians, and physicians at the conference generally accepted the distinction between the disciplined studies that make up the humanities and the process of being humanized; everyone was acquainted with people who excelled in the humanities but were unappealing as human beings. Despite this, and although a minority concern was expressed that an overt attempt to hire teachers of the humanities by medical schools might only be an administrative sham to counteract growing public disillusionment with what some people have come to regard as an increasingly inhumane profession, the general feeling of the group was that the humanities should occupy a more prominent place in medical education and that subsequent considerations should be given as to how this should be accomplished.

Certainly—for whatever reasons—up until that time there had been minimal use of the humanities in examining and resolving health-related ethical problems of all sorts. Technical advances, from organ transplantation to eugenics, forced ethical matters into the laps of physicians, who often took moral decisions upon themselves, however unsophisticated and uninformed they might have been—particularly if the rest of society had chosen to ignore the issues. There were broad moral and ethical issues to be considered, such as, Under what conditions, if any, can we allow transplantation of an unpaired organ? What should be society's position on euthanasia and abortion? What proportion of our health budget will go to increasing the availability of expensive, life-saving procedures and devices and what proportion will be directed toward preventive medicine?

In the future, it was agreed then and remains true today, scholars of the humanities and social sciences must be more involved in discussing issues at these broad levels. In addition, it was recognized in 1971 that there are problems about individual patients which arise every day in the hospital wards and clinics; often the young doctor or student is forced to take a stance which may have more far-reaching ethical or philosophic implications than he or she imagines. It is particularly at this level that experience in participation and interaction with the humanities is needed; up until 1970, it had been minimal. At a few medical schools, ward rounds often included nonphysician faculty members with training in philosophy, sociology, and theology. During the past fifteen years there has been an explosion of interest in most medical schools in the United States in involving the social sciences and humanities in their curricula in appropriate ways. What was an educational rarity at the time of the Arden House conference in 1971 became accepted practice in 1985. Most of the recent dialogue between the humanists and medical educators has focused on issues at these two levels (that is, the broad philosophic and ward consultation levels) and, appropriately, the dialogue has emphasized the moral and ethical implications of medical science and medical practice.

There is another potentially fruitful and as yet largely unexplored area of mutual interest between the humanities and medicine; it is with this third area, which involves the personal development of the physician, that this essay is primarily concerned.

The goal of medical education is to turn out practitioners, and, once a person has gone into practice, medical education should prepare him or her for a sufficiently satisfying life so that he or she will not want to leave the patient-care situation. What satisfies the physician in family or general practice? What gets him or her up at odd hours? What thread can make such a person happy, when he or she must face birth and death, sickness, anxiety and grief, tremendous character weaknesses or strengths? I suggest that this thread has little to do with science directly but is a cultivated interest in human nature, an interest that may sometimes equal that of the artist.

Hemingway chased all over the world to find his apocalypse in the bullring; others went to Montmartre or Greenwich Village to engage real life. But aware and sensitive physicians can find it all in their practice. If their sensitivities have been sharpened in chasing symbols through *Moby-Dick,*[1] *A Light in August,*[2] *The Hollow Men,*[3] and *The Waste Land,*[4] they may be able to find that much more enrichment in their day-to-day life. Instead of escaping from death and suffering in a cold or cynical denial, they may learn about them from those people they call "patients." I believe the complete physician must, at some point, contemplate such things as the confrontation with horror; the relationship between comedy and tragedy; the role of suffering in human development; the history of the work ethic and what it may mean to be deprived of the capacity to work; the concept that emotional maturity is related to the acceptance of one's own death, that death is a part of life; the role of "indifference" in the professional bearing of the physician; the beauty intrinsic to a well-established personal or professional relationship; the idea of a profession; and the rights of patients. No one has a greater opportunity to be closer to human nature than does the physician. The man or woman who sees this and enjoys that closeness will stay in clinical medicine. The humanities can help broaden his or her sensitivities and deepen his or her insights. Possibly the most dramatic recent role models in this regard are William Carlos Williams, whose poetry was born of his patients' dialogue, and Robert Coles, whose efforts as a psychiatrist and writer are inextricably intertwined.

The primary function of the humanities could be to focus upon the individual physician and his or her personal growth, emphasizing the need to work around the central issue of motivation and the nature of the satisfactions of a service-oriented life. As medical students become more deeply enmeshed in their career, a wide variety of personal questions will present themselves. The appropriately sensitized teacher of the humanities can help students recognize that the questions exist and can help them develop their own answers.

At the risk of confusing the reader by introducing a bewildering array of subjects, it might be useful to illustrate the kinds of questions which have been raised in my mind during my own medical education, which officially began in 1956. In raising these questions I have sometimes proposed my own answers or have described pertinent educational experiences for the reader's consideration. Where this is done, my aim has been only to illustrate more clearly the potential value of an interaction with scholars of the humanities. My goal is not to convince readers that my current views on these matters should be theirs.

Some of the questions that have crossed my mind follow: What is our role as physicians regarding our patients? Can we simply be ourselves or should we at times play a role for our patients' benefit? How much authority should we claim? When we are confronted with a sick patient who views us as a superhuman being riding a white charger, should we force our humanity and the imperfections and ambiguities of our skills and knowledge upon the patient, or should we gracefully accept the role in which the patient has cast us? An interesting aspect of this issue is whether some patients will project different images of strengths and virtues for male physicians as compared with female physicians. If so, it emphasizes the sensitivity required of the physician to ascertain where he or she "is" in the patient's vision.

Most mature physicians are more aware of the magnitude of their ignorance as compared with the depth of their own knowledge; is it wise, then, not to manifest an air of confidence for the patient's sake? Confidence is not synonymous with certainty and is not incompatible with humility.

What are the "rights" of patients; what kinds of psychologic roles can we sometimes force upon them and what roles do some of them take regardless? We frequently hear of the person who when hospitalized is treated like an infant by the health team; laymen seldom realize that many aggressively independent individuals literally regress and become like little children when they get sick or think they are sick. The sensitive doctor needs to be able to make these distinctions.

How does a physician learn to deal compassionately with suffering and anxiety of all sorts? It is necessary to have the capacity in every instance, almost intuitively, to ask "How would I feel in such a setting?" This alone, however, is not sufficient. We physicians must indeed understand ourselves well enough to know how we would feel—and that means all the feelings we would feel—in situations in which our patients find themselves; but we must also have enough humility to realize that we cannot react blindly according to our knowledge of our own feelings and should appreciate that others might react differently.

Have we the right to make moral judgments about our patients, especially those with different life-styles? Have we a right to be a doctor to just certain kinds of people, or should we be constantly attempting to understand and become empathetic with different styles and groups? On what legitimate grounds may we decline to take care of a person who seeks our help?

What role does "indifference" play in the bearing of the physician? T. S. Eliot, in his play *The Confidential Clerk*,[5] seems to make this quality of indifference an essential ingredient in the personal growth of his major character; to my reading, this quality is the opposite of emotional involvement. What is the difference between empathy and sympathy? How can one be empathetic and indifferent at the same time, and what good are such reflections for the individual attempting to be a useful physician?

What are the significant elements of the doctor-patient relationship? Medical faculty and students frequently discuss a well-worked-up diagnostic problem or the careful unraveling of a fascinating epidemiologic puzzle and wide appreciation is given in a variety of ways to the exquisite surgical procedure. It is difficult for me to recall in my own education any development of the concept of the beauty and importance of the successfully established doctor-patient relationship. This relationship is a difficult matter indeed for a patient and a physician living in an ever more transient America, bereft of hometowns and a sense of permanency. There is a knack to establishing this working relationship, and it must be defined and developed if more effective human delivery of health care is to occur.

Once I have become proficient at my trade and primarily involved in dispensing the fruits of my expertise, what can I learn and where is my chance for growth? With the apparent decline of orthodox religions, people these days seldom talk about spiritual development, and personality development seems to be something one should worry about only in the so-called formative years. Most of us somehow have come to accept the idea that everything important about our psyche was settled before our second birthday, so why bother? Some students may fail to see various possibilities if the process of medical education does not emphasize and capitalize upon the almost unique opportunity physicians have to work on their own development through their daily interaction with the gravest human personal problems. It is appalling to reflect upon the number of people, including physicians, who do not recognize that the basis for modern restlessness, ennui, and dissatisfaction is a deep and almost universal quest for individual meaning. Viktor Frankl, the famous psychiatrist who has written so compellingly on this subject based on his own personal experiences in surviving Nazi concentration camps, has made this existential quest for meaning the basis for logotherapy, a new approach to psychotherapy.

Physicians, like everyone else, need periodic refreshment and redirection, a refixing of their eyes upon their goals. As a profession, perhaps we have been a little embarrassed to speak of these things. The quality that separates the best physicians from the others is the degree of their motivation and their job satisfaction; and that in turn means they have to find meaning in what they do, to enjoy working with people and their problems, their strengths, their weaknesses, and their responses to crises.

How do I deal with dying patients and those who feel they have no hope? It is commonplace now, but nonetheless true, to point out that one of the greatest American taboos is the subject of death. In my own mind, maturity implies a realistic personal confrontation and handling of the idea of one's own death. As Americans become more aware of this taboo and attempt to counteract it in their individual lives, we are also experiencing the dissolution of the national gestalt of perpetual progress toward an attainable, perfect, just, and bountiful society. Thus, as a nation and culture we are dealing with emptiness and potential meaninglessness while increasing numbers of us are attempting to deal with the concept of our individual deaths. I think these are two dimensions of the same subject. Recent literature on these two subjects illustrates how the humanities can offer much to the understanding of the physician, who, after all, will need to deal with patients wrestling with the prospect of death, dread, or great suffering on the one hand or with the implications of a meaningless existence on the other.

Aristotle believed that the theater, through the presentation of tragedy, was therapeutic for the audience, although Plato strongly disagreed with this view and left no place for the poet in his Republic. In a recent book, literary scholar Stephen Booth comes down on Aristotle's side and in an interesting analysis tells why King Lear and Macbeth are good for you if you are in the audience. Elisabeth Kübler-Ross' book, *On Death and Dying, What the Dying Have to Teach Doctors, Nurses, Clergy and Their Own Families,*[6] has passages in it which seem analogous to ideas expressed by Michael Novak, the American philosopher and theologian, in his book *The Experience of Nothingness,*[7] which deals with the apparent meaninglessness of twentieth-century existence. Kübler-Ross makes a strong case for the prospect of personal growth through an effective confrontation with the concept of death rather than perpetuating the denial of death and suffering. Similarly, Michael Novak speaks about recognizing dealing with the "experience of nothingness" and contends that by refusing to run away from it or deny its existence, the individual personality may be taking the first step to a creative synthesis of individual personality and meaningful existence in the modern world. Mr. Novak says, "The experience of nothingness is an incomparably fruitful starting place for ethical inquiry. It is a vaccine against the lies upon which every civilization, the American civilization in particular, is built."

What is this experience of which Novak speaks and which he feels we Americans tend to deny as readily as we have denied death? He says it is a personal experience closely akin to the experiences of feelings about the meaninglessness of existence brought to the world's attention by people like Camus, Kierkegaard, and Sartre and illustrated most recently by the Theater of the Absurd. A quote from interesting television personality Dick Cavett describes at least a portion of the experience.

> I'm at my worst when I come out of a nap, and I can see with some kind of crystal clarity the existential absurdity of life. You can never do one-millionth of what's available. There's a sense of lassitude and emptiness about it all. And there's a clarity about it, which doesn't last very long, when I think, oh God, it isn't worth it. It's almost like seeing life from a photograph in the planetarium, where the earth is a small thing in all that space.

Perhaps part of Mr. Cavett's appeal is that his viewing audience recognizes this perspective in him and more and more Americans are finding it in themselves.

Of interest in this regard is an inscription apparently found in what was a burial ground for ancients well before the time of Christ. The inscription read, "I was not. I was. I am not. I don't care."

Kübler-Ross classifies the experience of dealing with death as she has recognized it among her patients roughly as follows (and it is of interest to substitute Novak's "experience of nothingness" for "death"): Step one: the abyss of death (or the experience of nothingness); step two: despair or depression; step three: there is no disintegration of the psyche and the issue has been faced; step four: the individual realizes he has faced it and it hasn't ruined him and his own courage gives him a sense of dignity and achievement. The latter must be akin to what I saw in my little daughter's eyes one day when she was so proud at having come down a big slide she had never previously had the courage to negotiate. In a very real sense, people who face death (or the experience of nothingness) accept it and have the courage to proceed with whatever else remains to them. They have conquered it. They develop a dignity others recognize. They have done what the astronauts appear to have done, they have dealt with the prospect of being blasted into infinity and have accepted that fate as a real possibility. Although it may in fact be true that some astronauts are fearless because they are among the world's best at denying death (it can't happen to me!), it is possible that in large measure they are such popular heroes because most of us transfer our own fears to them and assume that these men and women have dealt with death and have in fact conquered its fear.

Whether or not one shares Dr. Kübler-Ross' or Mr. Novak's ideas, it should be clear that the perceptions of people like them can be significant and stimulating elements in the continuing education of the developing physician.

What is nonverbal communication and which of its modalities are most likely to be useful to a health care worker? As physicians mature, they can learn more and more about this interesting area and can develop competence and pride in their abilities to communicate in a meaningful way with an increasingly greater variety of people. The white Anglo-Saxon Protestant presents a different problem in communication for the physician than does the hippie, the Native American, the black, the aged Irish Catholic, the Hispanic, the Gypsy, the Orthodox Jew, the paranoid individual, the stray or maverick, or the tracheotomized quadriplegic. There is much to be learned from artists and writers in this difficult matter of making a personal connection and I believe my own attempts at understanding some of the elements of novels by writers like Henry James, Virginia Woolf, and Dostoevsky have been helpful to me in later years as a physician. Jamake Highwater, artist and critic, has made the point that the fundamental objective, conscious or subconscious, of the artist is to communicate that which is within from his or her aloneness to other people; and he likens the effort to the intermittent blinking of stars trying to connect with others, galaxies and millennia away.[8] Hearing him speak of artists in this way, I could not help but be reminded of the dramatic aloneness experienced by people facing serious illness and the prospect of death. Mr. Highwater's lecture on this subject had the effect upon me (and other physicians in his audience) of broadening our perspective and understanding of patients, a subject that could not have been further from the lecturer's mind at that particular moment.

Parenthetically, I have come to believe that attempts to come to grips with artistic works of all sorts aid the physician in developing the kind of sensitivity to the patient that will enhance the ability to decipher the verbal and nonverbal messages that are conveyed. The visual and performing arts are after all attempts at communication, usually of emotions and perceptions, precisely the skills area in which an increasing number of patients find many modern doctors most deficient. Thus one might predict that noncompulsory, open university–type programs in the arts will find their way into medical schools on a regular basis over the next decade.

Patients can be helpful, too. I can recall an experience with a severely psychotic hospitalized patient whom I saw as a fourth-year medical stu-

dent over a two-month period. We met for an hour three times a week
and I still frequently reflect on some of the lessons she taught me. The
patient was a gigantic black lady in her mid thirties who had earned her
Ph.D. at a leading university and possessed an extraordinary intellect.
On top of her massive six-foot frame she had trained her hair so that it
rose upward from her head somewhat grotesquely an additional ten to
twelve inches. Her speech was apparently unintelligible, her language
symbolic, and people thought her to be hallucinating. Her eyes sought
out direct contact and I felt her to be challenging me to figure out what
she was saying; she seemed to be rejoicing at the perplexity and confusion of those of us who tried ever so intently and compulsively to interpret her ramblings. She seemed happy to enjoy these victories over
smaller intellects.

After each session I would review what had happened with the teaching psychiatrist whose practice and major interest were primarily with
schizophrenics. As the weeks wore on he got more excited about the fact
that I was making unusual progress with her and that she was telling me
more and more about what was bothering her most deeply. Intermingled
with unintelligible babbling, one could piece together a story she was
telling about a great ancestral princess, from some wondrous primordial
tribe, who got lost as an infant among a wild bunch of lesser beings and
who was forced to grow up amongst these sometimes well-meaning but
clearly inferior beasts. One day the princess' true father, a great king
and possibly god, came amongst the barbarians, identified his daughter,
anointed her in some way, and placed a tremendous crown upon her
head. None of the lesser creatures were aware of the meaning of all this
or of the princess' greatness, and they continued to think of her as an
ugly stranger. All this came out over two or three sessions amidst bab-
blings and ramblings delivered at the wall and ceiling but not at me.
Suddenly she stopped and looked directly at me and asked, "Do you
understand?" and for the first time she waited for an answer. For some
reason I said, "Yes, you are that princess; your hair is your crown; the
rest of us are the barbarians. But I want you to know that I respect you."
And I did respect her! I must have been right, because from that turning
point she seemed to speak more directly and honestly and formed the
beginnings of some kind of human relationship. It is even possible that
all of this did her some good. It certainly helped me in my pilgrimage.

Not all patients are so cryptic, but in order for the primary therapeutic physician-patient relationship to become established the patient must
learn, in some way or other, that the physician accepts the patient in a
nonjudgmental way and accords that patient a necessary and basic human respect. Once this has been achieved I believe there are then at least
three important messages to get across to the patient. To the extent that I

can convey these points successfully to the patient and to the extent that I live up to them is the measure (aside from the crucial matter of the quality of the technical medical ability and knowledge brought to bear on the case) of my success in achieving an effective therapeutic relationship with that particular patient. Here are three important messages which may or may not be delivered by explicit oral statements:

> I, as a physician, accept personal responsibility for you as a patient. I will do all I can to find out what is wrong with you and get you the best available treatment. If I can't find out or am confused in any way, I shall seek consultation and help from others. If you develop a fatal disease, I will stand by you and do all that is possible to minimize suffering and pain.

Once physicians understand the reality of this basic underpinning of the most creative kind of doctor-patient relationship, they can begin to explore at a conscious level whether they are well suited to deal with all patients or whether some patients will be more difficult or impossible for them. If they can't look a badly burned or disfigured or quadriplegic or dying patient in the eye and make this kind of commitment, then they shouldn't attempt to be that patient's primary physician.

> I, as a physician, wouldn't recommend anything for you as a patient that I wouldn't do for myself or my immediate family under the same circumstances.

Implicit in this message is the principle that the patient shapes or participates in the critical decisions involving his or her care. The patient may elect to delegate these decisions entirely to the physician or he or she may need to participate more actively in the decision-making process. For better or for worse (and I think it's for better), physicians are having to deal more and more frequently with patients who demand full participation in the crucial elements of their care.

> I, as the physician, am not emotionally involved with you as the patient.

Implicit here is a guarantee of scientific objectivity, a steady hand in surgery, a clear mind in diagnosis.

As an intern, I cared for an extraordinary man who came into our hospital for cardiac catheterization studies and evaluation for possible cardiac surgery. He was over sixty years of age, lean, muscular, hardworking, honest, kind, and tough. He had come to Montana many years

before with nothing and had worked up to ownership of a huge and productive farm. He was very proud of his children, all of whom had received magnificent educations. His respect for education seemed to me
to be not that of the average hard-working fellow who had missed the
college experience but rather came from a deep, intuitive philosophic
love for knowledge.

Five years before coming to us, his heart failed so that he couldn't
work any more, a condition completely unacceptable to him. When doctors at several medical centers refused to recommend surgery and in essence told him to learn to live with it, he went to the east coast where he
successfully went through a dangerous heart operation. He had won the
gamble and had returned to work. Now his heart was failing badly again,
but incredibly he had worked for ten hours on his tractor the day before
coming to our hospital for evaluation. I lived through the tests with him
and helped him interpret the findings and their implications. In essence,
they were as follows: no operation, little chance of improvement, and a
probable gradual downhill course with a sedentary existence versus dramatic open-heart surgery with a 50 percent operative mortality but a
reasonable chance of significant improvement if he survived the hospital
stay. Without batting an eyelash he chose surgery and returned to Montana to get a few things in order. I admired him immensely.

Some days later when he returned to the hospital under the care of
other physicians I went to the surgery ward to wish him well with the
operation the following morning. When I walked into the room he suddenly began to cry; I barely made it from the room without breaking down
similarly. Outside I did cry openly and I understood then that it was
good that I was no longer one of his physicians and would not be called
upon to help in his surgery. I learned from this experience about the
quality of "indifference," something I couldn't quite learn from reading
T. S. Eliot's *The Confidential Clerk*. The trick is to care but to be indifferent; that is, not emotionally involved. It is not always possible.

Although my tears were inappropriate because they were really for me
and I didn't die, the man had cried appropriately, for he never regained
consciousness after surgery.

I am not suggesting that my positions on these proposed elements of
the doctor-patient relationship are the right ones or the only ones, but I
am suggesting that the concerned physician must come to grips with
these questions, and that artists, performers, and humanities teachers
may be helpful in aiding each maturing physician in developing his or
her own particular answers.

It seems embarrassingly self-evident to me that physicians in training
should be continually exposed to this type of analysis and thinking or

else they will be painfully inadequate as they try to understand the world in which they live. I believe that one of the challenges to medical education in the immediate future is to learn how best to implement this proposed interaction of the arts, the humanities, and medicine so that the students are engaged on their own grounds. It will not be an easy challenge to meet.

## Notes

1. H. Melville, *Moby-Dick; or The Whale* (Chicago: Encyclopaedia Britannica, 1952).

2. W. Faulkner, *Light in August* (New York: Random House, 1932).

3. T. S. Eliot, "The Hollow Men," in *Collected Poems, 1909–1962* (New York: Harcourt, Brace and World, 1963), 51–76.

4. Eliot, "The Waste Land," in ibid., 79–82.

5. T. S. Eliot, *The Confidential Clerk,* in *The Complete Plays of T. S. Eliot* (New York: Harcourt, Brace and World, 1963), 217–291.

6. E. Kübler-Ross, *On Death and Dying* (New York: Macmillan, 1969).

7. M. Novak, *The Experience of Nothingness* (New York: Harper and Row, 1970).

8. J. Highwater, from the Betty Wheless Trotter Lectures, University of Texas Health Science Center, Houston, Texas, 1984.

# 18. *A Postscript from the Physician as Patient: Some Observations on Having a Coronary*

**David E. Rogers**

I've just spent what is for me quite an unusual ten minutes. I've been looking at flowers. Obviously I've seen flowers all of my life. In recent years my wife's interest in plants has led me to learn more about them. But until right now I have never really appreciated their vivid coloring, or their intricate design, or the exquisite shaping of their petals, or stamens, or foliage, or just how delicately they are put together. I had never taken the time necessary to just *indulge* in them. I can report that I found it most pleasurable.

So that's the teaser. I hope it suggests that I am enjoying life and savoring it. But I'm using it as a lead-in to something else. As a doctor who has spent much of his professional lifetime trying to listen very carefully to patients and to treat them appropriately and then to teach others who are becoming doctors how to do it well, a recent experience prompts me to try to describe what one very common disease feels like "from the inside" when it starts.

The disease is commonplace—a myocardial infarction.

This peculiarly human disease probably appeared quite suddenly
on the historical scene sometime toward the end of the nineteenth and
the early part of the twentieth century. After its recognition it rapidly
zoomed to the number one position on the mortality hit list in much of
the western world. In this country it reached its apogee in 1963. Since
then it seems to have been becoming both less common and somewhat
more benign.

Clearly, what I have to say here will not add to anyone's understanding
of this number one killer of American men of middle age. However, my
pedagogical instincts are hard to control, and several young doctors who
have quizzed me about what it feels like have suggested I try to put the
sensations—not the pathology—into words while the experience is still
vivid. I think this suggestion was made in part so that they could be
spared yet further verbal details from me and get about their more pressing business. However, I promised them I would try.

I will omit all the details about what I was doing or the prodrome
(which was classic) and will simply try to describe the episode itself,
for soon after its onset I knew precisely what was happening to me and I
had quite an amount of time to think about it.

I have often told medical students that most people I've queried who
are having genuine cardiac pain seem to instinctively wish to remain
very quiet even when their pain is not particularly severe. Thus, I've generally felt that chest pain is probably noncardiac when patients have told
me they've had to keep "wiggling about" to find a comfortable position
or were "writhing with pain" and the like.

My own experience would certainly confirm this. After the first fifteen to twenty minutes, when the pain was waxing and waning and I was
pretending it was esophageal and popping a few antacids and drinking a
glass of milk, the pain certainly told me just what it seems to have told
other patients. I felt I must sit down *very, very* quietly. Despite doing
so, the pain became a steadily expanding deep penetrating ache spread-
ing from beneath mid breast bone, around the sides of my chest, up my
neck into my lower jaw, and down the inner aspect of my left arm into
my fourth and fifth fingers. It would cycle a bit. Sometimes it would
seem most dreadful in my chest, then in my jaw and lower teeth, then in
my left arm. But it had one clear message. What I felt from the outset
and continued to feel through about two hours of what seemed absolutely intolerable pain was that if I remained *absolutely* immobile, not
moving even an eyelash, perhaps it would let go of me. I would guess it
took about ten to twelve minutes to build to maximal intensity and there
it stayed. During the entire period I sat absolutely still with my eyes
closed, conscious of the fact that I was sweating profusely and that I
probably looked very pale and very lousy. Although my wife was bus-

tling cheerfully around in the kitchen not fifteen feet away, I said absolutely nothing, feeling that even moving my tongue or vocal chords was simply too much. There was no inclination to groan or cry out.

There was another aspect of the pain frequently alluded to by others. There was absolutely no doubt in my mind that I was about to die. As the pain remained, I simply wished exodus would go ahead and happen. The emotion I can recapture regarding this certainty was not one of great fear but rather of anger mixed with sadness. Anger that this goddamned thing was happening to me and the knowledge that I had done some things—years of smoking and some more recent episodes of handling stress rather poorly—which had provoked it. Sadness that I wasn't going to be able to say goodbye to anybody, particularly my family and close friends and colleagues, or tell them what they had meant to me.

The quality of the pain is as difficult for me to describe as it seems to have been for other observers over the last seventy plus years. It was not the bright or burning or well-localized pain one feels with a cut or a puncture or a burn from which one instinctively and swiftly retreats. A very different set of nerve endings is involved. It was a dreadful, deep, nauseating ache. If you could multiply one hundred–fold the kind of ache in your arms you experience after working too long with them trying to screw in a recalcitrant light bulb in a ceiling socket that is a little too high over your head to reach decently, you'll be close. The stunt I tried many years ago—of putting a blood pressure cuff on my own leg above the knee, blowing it up to occlude arterial circulation, and then feeling the kind of pain which appears in one's calf (which quickly becomes pretty dreadful)—is yet closer (I was trying to see if I could mimic heart pain). But what was exquisitely different about that situation is that I could release the cuff when I felt I could not stand further intensity of pain. In this instance there was no such letup.

As to intensity, I keep wanting to use the word "unbearable," but obviously this wasn't true any more than was my certain conviction that I would die. But it was an absolutely monstrously awful sensation and it was totally untouched by twenty or thirty or forty milligrams of morphine given me over the next two hours. That morphine gave so little relief has made me feel for the hundreds of patients with the same disease I've treated with this drug.

So that's what it feels like. To simply put some finishing touches on the nice ending which obviously makes this self-serving introspection possible, let me add yet a few more comments.

First, having a cardiac catheterization via femoral artery and vein during an infarction is a piece of cake. Almost no discomfort. Further, frequent squirts of dye into one's coronaries, which I could watch on the monitor, is totally without unpleasant sensation. It did not improve my morale to see absolutely no dye going into my left anterior descending coronary, which appeared completely blocked, but I already knew that this was probably going to be the case, and all other arteries looked splendid.

One further episode was impressive and of profound relief to me. My cardiologist catheter artisans had maneuvered their catheter into the stumplike orifice of the left anterior descending and begun dripping in streptokinase (an ancient streptococcal enzyme I first used in crude form to dissolve clots in pleural spaces in 1950). Quite suddenly, and after only modest amounts of enzyme, I said—and I think these were some of my first words since onset—"I think you've dissolved it, I've lost my pain." They were quite surprised, but they shot in some more dye which confirmed part of what I was saying. A thin threadlike squirt of dye could be seen going through a very tight inch-long obstruction close to the origin of the coronary. But the whole artery below the block could be seen looking fat and filled. They continued to profuse the streptokinase, but five to ten minutes later I said, "And now it's clotted off again," for my pain had just then returned in its original intensity. More pictures showed that this indeed was true—no more filling beyond the stump.

Then followed the use of the latest in modern medical miracle technologies. My colleagues skillfully threaded a tiny wire through the obstruction, guided a collapsed balloon over it, and positioned it within the inch-long obstruction. This I watched on the monitor with fascination. Then they expanded the balloon, forcing arterial wall, clot, and atheroma outward. Again, swift and blissful relief of pain. They measured pressures and gradients, fooled around, and inflated it again a few times over the next thirty to forty minutes to make sure the gradient had been eliminated and that it didn't clot off again, and I have been pain free ever since. Subsequent pictures of the coronary looked virtually normal.

Let me describe just one other thing which my physicians did for me later, for I have felt, in retrospect, that it was a vital factor in speeding my return to full function. Although I had been agitating to get home, I will now confess to some feelings of apprehension about it while still in the hospital. Being hooked up to all that gadgetry makes one feel surprisingly dependent and fragile and emotionally uncertain about one's ability to function adequately outside the hospital's technological womb. Thus, I had some doubts about how I would feel walking up the stairs or up the driveway and the like.

But the night before discharging me, my cardiologists asked if I would like them to run a modified stress test on me before I left, and I agreed with enthusiasm. Consequently, the next morning they hooked me up, stuck me on the treadmill, and proceeded to work me until I thought I would drop. My legs were crying for relief and I was puffing like an aging bull, but my electrocardiogram remained totally unchanged, my blood pressure behaved responsibly, and I had absolutely no chest pain. Afterward I felt that this was perhaps the greatest gift they could have bestowed upon me as a going-away present. Although I was intellectually sure my heart was functioning splendidly, to have objective proof that it could handle vastly more effort than I was planning for it during the next month or so made me feel totally comfortable about cutting the umbilical cord and striking out on my own again.

So I have had an experience unheard of until very recently—that of knowing first-hand what having a massive myocardial infarction feels like, but without it actually occurring or without having to live with its crippling aftermath. The residual damage looks modest and should repair rapidly. My coronaries are now all good-looking garden hoses without obstruction. And perhaps of equal long-term significance, my priorities have been abruptly but quite appropriately reordered. Thus, my leisurely and pleasurable look at the flowers.

My last observation: as we continue to struggle to make medical care less expensive without lousing it up, I am obviously going to be thinking hard about the implications of what I have just experienced.

First, I would guess that within a very few years it may be viewed as close to medical malpractice to hospitalize a patient with an acute evolving coronary anywhere but in a hospital with a cardiac unit with catheterization, angioplasty, and backup surgical capabilities, unless such a unit is more than two hours away. That sure as hell won't reduce acute costs.

But as some of my vintage colleagues and I have since said to each other, we used to care for people like me by slugging them with morphine until their blood-starved heart muscle died and their pain stopped. We would watch fairly helplessly when they developed fatal arrhythmias. We agonized about giving them digitalis when they went into congestive heart failure because of its propensity to produce fatal arrhythmias and it sometimes did. Our patient stayed in the hospital for a minimum of six weeks (I stayed ten days) and we created a dreadful number of cardiac cripples who never worked productively again.

So obviously it's a no contest trade-off as far as I'm concerned, although you might recognize a certain personal bias in that point of view. As one of my trustee-doctor-surgeon colleagues is fond of saying, "Sometimes the best medicine is the most expensive medicine." All I can say is "Amen" in this instance, but over the long haul, it seems pretty cost beneficial to me!

# 19. *A Dialogue with Hippocrates and Griff T. Ross, M.D.*

**Roger J. Bulger**

Once every century, Hippocrates is allowed to leave the Elysian fields to interview a physician deemed most characteristic of the Hippocratic essence. For the twentieth century he was sent to visit with Dr. Griff Ross, a fourth-generation family physician in Mount Enterprise, Texas. Dr. Ross left his practice in this small east Texas town to join the armed forces during World War II. He returned to a Mayo Clinic residency and became an internationally known reproductive endocrinologist and career scientist at the National Institutes of Health. His last job at NIH was as deputy director of the Clinical Center. Dr. Ross then returned to Texas to become associate dean for clinical affairs at the University of Texas Medical School at Houston, whereupon his genius as a teacher and inspirer of students and faculty alike came to full bloom. The last years, and particularly the last several months, of Dr. Ross' life were painful because of an almost incredible battle with cancer, during which Dr. Ross and his doctors attacked the disease vigorously and at every opportunity.

Hippocrates and Dr. Ross sat on the porch of the Ross family home in Mount Enterprise one warm July evening in 1985.

HIPPOCRATES: Good evening, Dr. Ross! It's a great privilege for me to meet with you.

DR. ROSS: Good evening, Dr. Hippocrates. Indeed it is my honor to . . .

HIPPOCRATES: Please, Dr. Ross, no "doctor" before my name. We didn't use any special terms in my day, believing that the fruits of our labors earned us honor that no title could bestow. In fact, you can call me anything, except perhaps Hippo—it sounds so . . . Roman!

DR. ROSS: I am terribly honored to have been chosen to have this opportunity to talk with you, but I still cannot fathom why I've been selected . . .

HIPPOCRATES: We have our reasons!

DR. ROSS: . . . unless it is in part because I spent a lot of time talking with my friend Roger Bulger about a book, *In Search of the Modern Hippocrates,* that he is preparing for publication. We talked a lot about what you would say or think regarding the material he chose to include in the book. I'd be delighted if we could use that book and its various essays as a starting point for our discussions, because it contains what we thought a twenty-first-century Hippocrates would have to deal with.

HIPPOCRATES: That's more than agreeable to me, Dr. Ross. You know, we have an astounding pre-print service in the Elysian fields, so I've read the book in detail and with great interest. I must say that some of the ideas and observations appeal more to me than others, but it's also true that I don't know much about your modern western society and by nature am remote from much of it. In fact, I am certain of very little even from my own time. What we knew for a fact four hundred years before Christ was so miniscule in comparison to what was guesswork or intuition.

DR. ROSS: Well, we also know far less than what we don't know. And what we do "know" as based in reasonable scientific observation is generally highly provisional. On the other hand, what is so exciting about 1985 is that we are continuing to learn at such a tremendous rate.

HIPPOCRATES: True. Clearly the fifty-year period preceding 1985 has been the most scientifically productive in history. You have a great deal to be proud of. We estimate that 95 percent of all the scientists in the history of the human race were alive in 1985. But people and nations and cultures are sometimes strangely perverse; just when you have made such enormous strides you seem to be doubting your science and withdrawing your support, relatively speaking.

DR. ROSS: You speak as though that's your major concern about us.

HIPPOCRATES: It is in the long-term sense. Your western society seems to be losing faith in the truth, both truth speaking and truth seeking—a peculiar cynicism indeed. It is ultimately a cynicism about the prospects for a viable future. One has to worry about a society with diminishing concern for its children and its children's children.

DR. ROSS: I'd like to pursue that discussion in depth, Hippocrates, but I can't stand the suspense of waiting to hear what your major short-term or immediate concern is for modern medicine.

HIPPOCRATES: Oh, that's an easy question and the concern is a very real one based upon our Elysian fields opinion pollsters. We can keep track on a minute-to-minute basis of people's opinions regarding important matters because our equipment registers every major thought immediately as it formulates itself coherently in the individual human brain.

DR. ROSS: Wow! As we used to say in Mount Enterprise, Texas, when I was growing up, that kind of technology could get you into tall grass in a hurry!

HIPPOCRATES: Well, we didn't have any tall grass on Cos, so I don't know what you mean by that, but I do know that in 1985, for the first time in millennia, doctors are actively discouraging their own children from entering the profession. This is not an isolated phenomenon or a minor movement. It is so widespread that only a small minority of doctors are categorically advocating medicine to their children as a great and honored profession of which it is a great privilege to be a member.

DR. ROSS: I can grant your point, but I hadn't realized it was so widespread a feeling among today's doctors.

HIPPOCRATES: That's because Harris hasn't included it in his poll yet, but that's coming. The sad thing is that the dentists have already convinced lots of the best young folks who had been entering dentistry even a few years ago not to do so, and I am afraid that will happen in medicine, too.

DR. ROSS: But why do you suppose this is happening? Aren't we really at the height of our performance and effectiveness as a healing profession?

HIPPOCRATES: I am grieved to say that the issue is money and to a lesser extent independence, freedom, and what you all call accountability.

DR. ROSS: Please explain.

HIPPOCRATES: Well, from where I sit (which after all does provide a broad perspective), doctors in America have become too successful financially. So many of them have to spend too much time worrying about how to spend or keep their money that it actually diminishes their doctoring. The worst thing, now that you've gotten me on the subject, is the preferential reimbursement for techniques and procedures. That has encouraged many doctors to become more procedure than patient oriented.

The upshot is that doctors will be earning less and are feeling a grow-

ing disapprobation from the public. The society is bureaucratizing medicine and in the interest of "accountability" many onerous procedures are
being forced on the profession, and that is depressing to existing practitioners. Furthermore, most doctors in America now are private independent practitioners and have always enjoyed the potential of moving
virtually anywhere to do their thing. Just a few years ago a good person
could get into any specialty in any location. Now, all that's changed.

Choices are shrinking at every level. The overproduction of doctors
will fuel the rapid switch to group practice, often in salaried situations,
increasingly in organizations neither owned nor managed by the doctors.
All these forces, I think, are creating a situation which is frankly worrisome to even the very best of mature practitioners, especially when it
comes to encouraging good young people to enter medicine.

DR. ROSS: But, what to do about all that? What's wrong with this prevailing view? Isn't it a realistic response to an all-too-true set of circumstances? What will happen to the profession if the best and brightest stop
choosing it? What will the future bring? You must know!

HIPPOCRATES: So many questions, Dr. Ross! I see I touched an area of
concern for you too.

. DR. ROSS: Indeed you have. But do tell me. Will our profession go
downhill in the next generation? Has the golden age passed?

HIPPOCRATES: I can't tell you. Of course, I know the answers to your
questions, but part of the ground rules of these conversations is that I
cannot inform you about what to you is in the future. It is up to you to
find out in due course on your own.

DR. ROSS: Well then, can you at least tell me how you would react if
you were in our situation?

HIPPOCRATES: That I can do. First of all, we need to be realistic,
practical, and observing of the facts and not particularly mindful of hypotheses about the future which may or may not come about. Every age
has its doomsayers and its mass or group moods. I would try to identify
what is good and creative about the profession and try to implement and
preserve those characteristics.

For example, I'm not sure that I share all of Dr. Relman's views (chapter 15) about the medical-industrial complex, but I totally agree with his
most important point that doctors individually and as a group should divest themselves of financial interests in health-related businesses which
would leave them open to financial conflict of interest charges vis-à-vis
the main concern of the doctor as the patient's major advocate.

I like what Dr. Reiser (chapters 12 and 16) has to say about future
technology actually providing the doctor more time to talk with the patient. Jay Katz, in his recent book on informed consent, *The Silent World
of Doctor and Patient*, emphasizes the need for what he terms "conver-

sation" between doctor and patient. Dr. Reiser and Dr. Bulger (chapters 12 and 8) have emphasized the power of words and communication in general to create an environment in which the patient, nature's own recuperative powers, and the doctor's interventions can come together to produce maximal benefit for the patient. Aspects of this main point of listening and talking are essential dimensions of the essays by Erikson, Majno, Coles, and Spiro (chapters 5, 10, 11, and 13). There is such a thing as a healing relationship.

DR. ROSS: As Richards points out in his essay, for most of the past two thousand years, and especially in the last one hundred years, we have been trying to conquer and to control nature, to defeat death, our seemingly implacable enemy. But recently I've noticed another trend growing, and that is the desire to control and to gain mastery over the technologies we've invented to control nature! Along with this has come an awareness of our cultural denial of death, the virtual taboo status of the subject of death in our society. This is leading to an awareness of the need to more fully inform our patients, to let them control their own destinies, and to be scrupulously honest with them. There are those who argue that these behavioral elements are essential to the basic trust so crucial to the development of the healing relationship you just mentioned.

HIPPOCRATES: Spoken like a Greek, Dr. Ross! And the other side of that coin, which I hate to say remains reasonably characteristic of many physicians' behaviors, is the sense of abandonment felt by the patient of a doctor who refuses to discuss death and dying, who by implication regards it as a hostile act on the part of the patient, who in turn will be punished by a turning away on the part of the doctor. Patients' friends and family then learn to interpret by extension all physician silence as abandonment. I think honesty and truth telling must be even more important in your transient, restless society, seemingly bereft of hometowns and permanent friendships. More and more people understand that scientifically validated treatments make up a surprisingly small percentage of the treatments currently considered standard in modern practice, and therefore the commitment to candor, truth telling, and truth seeking in your physicians is ever more essential to the successful practice of the art of scientific medicine.

DR. ROSS: Some of us have real trouble dealing with uncertainty; it's like dealing with death in some ways . . .

HIPPOCRATES: I guess, Dr. Ross, the bottom line of my advice to my twenty-first-century counterparts is that, especially in difficult times, it is best to get back to the basics, and it seems to me that there have been too many distractions from the basics of doctoring for the welfare of all concerned.

DR. ROSS: What about the emphasis on dealing creatively with suffer-

ing and death, which is a prominent part of the book? I know Dr. Bulger
has worried about its prominence.

HIPPOCRATES: Well, all that would have been unnecessary in my time,
because suffering and death were all around us. We could not escape for
such prolonged periods as you people have been able to. However, I
agree with the emphasis, because the doctor, to heal, must be willing to
stand by, to help in even the worst and most hopeless of circumstances
or else the patient cannot feel secure that he or she has a doctor. In America in 1985, where even a major war, famine, pestilence, or other disaster has been basically unknown to the population for so long, you are in
particular need of what my friend Aristotle used to advocate. Although
I didn't go in much for his prattling on about abstract subjects, I could
relate to his idea that the audiences viewing our Greek theatrical productions would benefit from a creative emotional catharsis. So much the
more so for your contemporary population and your students and doctors, because untimely death and suffering have touched them so seldom. I agree that the writings of the poets and philosophers and the
visions of the artists, while helpful in any age, should be especially
helpful to you people in dealing emotionally and intellectually with
suffering.

Parenthetically, although I greatly admire your anesthesia, it grieves
me greatly whenever I hear of an anesthetic death in someone seeking to
escape what really amounts to relatively minor pain. So unnecessary! It
almost seems to us that you in America are seeking a pain-free environment for life!

DR. ROSS: But doesn't that relate to the so-called cultural boredom we
have experienced which expresses itself as a lack of personal meaning to
the individual?

HIPPOCRATES: I guess so, although I cannot relate in my bones to cultural boredom and meaninglessness. All I know is that I would give my
eye teeth to have lived in a time and society such as yours with such tremendous opportunities and with things happening so fast. In comparison,
things were so boring in my day . . . oops!

DR. ROSS: You see!

HIPPOCRATES: Well, maybe I do know about boredom, but life was so
tenuous and generally so short that since death could come at any instant we seemed to fight to get each extra day of life. But, to get to the
crux of your interest, I do think the essays dealing with suffering and
death are on target and important.

By the way, I would like to put in a plug for logotherapy, that new
thrust led by Dr. Viktor Frankl of Vienna. It addresses the suffering
issue best and offers the physician some therapeutic options even in
the most difficult cases. I could never buy Freud's view that the sexual

drive ruled human life, nor could I accept Adler's concept that the will to power governed behavior. I am much more comfortable with the concept that the will to meaning is the universal characteristic that encompasses us all.

DR. ROSS: I thought you started by saying you couldn't relate in your bones to the concept of meaninglessness.

HIPPOCRATES: Obviously I misspoke or was guilty of faulty thinking.

DR. ROSS: It's amazing how readily you admit error!! I guess some people could find or seek their meaning by fulfilling their sexual drives or by expressing their will to power . . .

HIPPOCRATES: Yes, but Frankl's view is that to provide meaning to an individual life a goal must be self-transcendant; that is, aimed at something the individual perceives as being beyond his or her immediate self-gratification. And that, I think, would be helpful to your society if it could catch on more widely as a way of looking at things. By the way, doctoring offers just such a goal for self-fulfillment, which is why I would be hopeful that some of the very best young people would always seek to enter our field.

DR. ROSS: In a very real way, a major aim of the book is to encourage young people to continue to seek careers in medicine. That's why I personally am a little worried about the book's emphasis on lying and honesty. It seems a little gratuitous for the general reader.

HIPPOCRATES: Gratuitous only to those already committed to honesty. I can attest to the fact that lying and deceit are the scourge of every age. So I vote to keep those essays that deal with placebos, lying, and the pursuit of honesty in a prominent place in the book. I found stimulating the differing perspectives of Spiro, Reiser, Crawshaw, and Bulger. Naturally, I liked the emphasis on Socrates' life and found it very accurate indeed.

I think that striving for absolute honesty is so important to the would-be healer that any purposeful compromise should not be encouraged. Clearly Dr. Spiro and others are supportive of placebos under certain circumstances and, at least on the surface, seem to be favoring purposeful deception of the patient, even if only rarely.

I don't think we should purposely deceive any patient, but I do not believe you modern people have achieved the knowledge necessary to prove that giving a vitamin pill to an elderly individual who believes in vitamins and pills will not in fact release one or several helpful chemicals from that extraordinary pharmacy we all carry between our ears.

I think it would be wrong to give a chocolate drop to a patient while telling him or her this was a potent medicine which will cure his or her backache. But I don't think it would be wrong to prescribe any one of a number of pills, identifying them accurately to the patient, indicating that you have no scientific knowledge that this will help but that you as the physician believe that in this instance, in this patient, this pill might help the patient to cure himself or herself.

It seems to me there's a difference between offering a treatment modality even when there's no scientific evidence to support such an approach and adopting the view that we shall only offer treatments that have been scientifically proven. I believe that the placebo effect can be more widely utilized by a physician dealing honestly with patients with all the tools at his or her command than the odd attempt to deceive a patient about the efficacy of a pill.

DR. ROSS: You are saying that there's a common ground among those authors you mentioned. I agree with you and have often felt that the placebo is not a subject for discussion in and of itself. I think it is only a subset of the real subject, which is the role of emotions in the healing of disease and prevention of illness. I have been sick much of my recent adult life and during those experiences, if I do say so myself, I have had the opportunity to be as well informed about the science of medicine as virtually anyone I know. I have known the statistics and the odds, but I have also known that where there's life, there's hope and a chance to beat the odds. And I have done it, too. I recall once having a most difficult and trying hospitalization, wherein the tide of my illness turned upon, in my own mind, an unusual therapeutic experience. I had just been through the ordeal of waiting for several hours for a radiologic procedure in a truly inhumane and undignified setting with other humans crowded in various stages of dress and undress like sides of beef in a butcher's refrigerator. As I returned to my room on the elevator, my distress and anxiety must have been apparent to the black elevator operator who had become a friend. He suggested we drop to our knees and pray for my recovery. We did and I did! It was a truly therapeutic experience which for the nonreligiously inclined can now be conceived of in believable biochemical terms.

HIPPOCRATES: I hear you, Dr. Ross, and I agree. I offer the observation that one of the reasons you were chosen for this conversation arises from the fact that you have been so sick so many times in your adult life. You have never forgotten that the word physician means teacher and you have used your misfortunes to educate those around you in an extraordinary fashion.

DR. ROSS: Well, I've had a really bad time of it the past two years— enormous and repetitive sufferings, including the past four months in the hospital.

HIPPOCRATES: I know and many of your friends were quietly aghast at all the extraordinary efforts the doctors took to cure you. They thought you should have been allowed to die in peace and dignity.

DR. ROSS: And some of my friends weren't so quiet about that. They meant well but they underestimated me and my doctors. I've been in control of my treatment the whole way. I've been suffering and I know the chances get less and less, but each moment of life for me is of such value. My wife, Pinky, and I believe that not to try to preserve life is not to affirm it—and the suffering has been worth it. I know so many have visited and interacted with me—I have seen in their eyes the sorrow but also the wonder at what we were doing and in some the recognition of what my wife and I wished to live out. You know, when confronted with hard choices, sometimes you can only choose not to choose the ones you don't want.

Is there ever any use for a good joke on the Elysian fields?

HIPPOCRATES: Humor is always welcome, Dr. Ross. Tell me!

DR. ROSS: Well, it has seemed to me that my situation has been analogous to that of the little boy who agreed with his younger brother one night that they would use some bad words the next day to shock their mother, who was a strict, no-nonsense disciplinarian. Their strategy developed and they agreed that the younger boy would use the word "hell" and the older boy "ass." They shook hands on their pact and went to sleep contentedly. The next morning they went down to breakfast and the mother asked the younger boy whether he wanted Wheaties, Rice Crispies, or Cheerios in his bowl. The young boy paused and said, "Oh, what the hell, I'll take the Cheerios!"

Whop! The punishment came swift and sure and devastatingly from the mother. The little boy was whimpering and the spilled Cheerios had been picked up when the mother turned to the older of the boys and asked which of the cereals he wanted.

Summoning his courage, he said, "Gosh, Mom, I don't know, but you can bet your sweet ass it won't be Cheerios!"

HIPPOCRATES: Ha, ha, ha . . . so you've used humor to help you deal with the reality of unpleasant choices!

DR. ROSS: I wouldn't recommend this route to everyone. You need the right wife and the right family. And in fact the suffering has been so great that I've despaired at times and wished it would end. The longer it has gone on, the more difficult it has been to find myself in this suffering and to understand who I am. But I know my role is to teach through example and I'm going to keep at it until the last breath.

HIPPOCRATES: You have just explained why you were chosen. You have lived so much of what Pellegrino and Erikson write about that you have exemplified for any aspiring modern Hippocrates the character they must have to best match the responsibilities they aspire to take on. Human relations skills, enormous integrity, and an understanding or willingness to deal with suffering and death must accompany the scientific talents and technical knowledge of what I would call the modern complete physician.

DR. ROSS: Could you comment on the historical and philosophic essays? Should they be a part of this book?

HIPPOCRATES: Gladly, Dr. Ross. Dickinson Richards, who was a truly great physician, scientist, and later student of my activities and those making up my followers, is unerringly accurate in his portrayal of me and the origin of the Hippocratic Oath. He is correct that I didn't write it and find it a bit more detailed and inflexible in certain areas than I would have liked, even in my own day. However, the primacy of the patient's interests and the sense of commitment that that ancient oath proclaims are points with which I concur completely. He is correct too in his description of our interest twenty-five hundred years ago in the environment, its impact on health, and the importance of people living in harmony with nature.

Now, as for that Dr. Pellegrino, he, I must say, says it all when I project what would seem important to me were I practicing in your modern world. You must understand that even after almost twenty-five hundred years in these Elysian fields I have not fully yielded my prejudices against the Romans for taking so much of our culture away. Despite this deficiency (and I am working on my personal prejudices), I must admit that, though he has a Roman name, Dr. Pellegrino thinks like a Greek philosopher. The primacy of competence in the physician's make-up is an essential message to send to the public in your increasingly impersonal, transient, and uncertain world; it implies a major commitment on the part of the doctor, for it is not as easy to maintain technical competence now as when I was working. A reliance on a growing personal clinical experience was really all that we had. In 1985 such a reliance, if unchecked by continuing efforts to keep up with alternate tests and treatments and if unaccompanied by a healthy sense of the uncertainty in distinguishing among competing approaches to therapy, can be very dangerous indeed. Pellegrino addresses group responsibilities and social contracts in significant fashions and I commend him for his essay.

Naturally, after all these centuries, I am particularly attuned to the impact of cultural differences on health, disease, and healing. Romanucci-Ross, Tancredi, and Majno are right on.

DR. ROSS: One of the questions Dr. Bulger and I have often discussed is if you were alive today and if you were to author a modern oath, what would your oath look like?

HIPPOCRATES: Oh, thank you! I thought you'd never ask! It happens I have a draft of a modern oath right here. Before I read it to you, you should know that I submitted it to the editor at the Elysian Fields Press. He thought the prose was all right for a doctor, but he indicated it wouldn't sell in 1985. It is too long and complicated and can't be easily tailored for television. He sent it to the marketing chief who fixed it, but I didn't accept their recommendations, so I'm afraid you won't like it.

DR. ROSS: Don't worry, Hippocrates; if I can convince people that you wrote it, they'll buy it. I'll need that marketing chief to help me convincingly demonstrate its authenticity. We might even spin off a for-profit subsidiary . . .

HIPPOCRATES: I hope that's a joke. One other point—I have a thing about words and names. I know it's the vogue now to refer to people seeking the physician's help as "clients" rather than as "patients"; the rationale behind this thrust is the laudable effort to redress the uneven balance in the relationship between doctor and patient and to emphasize the patient's primary role in deciding his or her own fate. I have used both terms, however. When the individual is sick or injured, for me he or she is a patient, because that word means sufferer; when the individual is not sick and seeks preventive services or advice of various sorts, he or she becomes a client, a term which came into our language referring to vassals relating to a feudal lord.

I apologize for these caveats and for being a little defensive about my new oath. You see, I've been working on it for years and it is, after all, the first oath I've ever written.

DR. ROSS: Your prefatory comments have been helpful, but I'm ready for the new oath.

HIPPOCRATES: The Modern Physician's Oath, 1985.

• I, as a physician, accept personal responsibility for the care of my patients and promise candor and a spirit of truthfulness in the faithful transmission of medical information. I will do all I can to find out what is wrong with each patient and to get him or her the best available treatment. If I can't find out or am confused in any way, I shall seek consultation and help from others. If the patient develops a fatal disease, I shall stand by him or her and do all that is possible to minimize suffering and pain.

• I, as a physician, shall recommend for each patient only those things I would like to have done for myself or my immediate family under the same circumstances.

• I, as a physician, recognize the fact that any patient's values may be different from mine and I accept each patient in a nonjudgmental way, according to each a full measure of basic human respect. I shall seek to involve all patients as fully as they wish in the decisions relating to their care and shall vigilantly seek to serve them in accordance with their values. If my patients' values are not consistent in any particular instance with the laws of our society, or if my own value system precludes my serving them in a particular way, or if any institutional commitment prevents me from placing their interests first, I shall so inform them and help them consider the options.

• I, as a physician, shall seek to become a friend to all my patients but shall not use my power to take advantage of them or to allow my feelings to intrude on my judgment and objectivity.

• I, as a physician, pledge to do my utmost to sustain my knowledge and skills at the highest possible level to assure professional competence at all times.

• I, as a physician, firmly believe in and am committed to the principle of the major role of the profession in quality assurance relating to the care rendered by individual doctors. Thus, I welcome participation in efforts by professional physician societies to improve health care and to monitor aspects of health care. I am dedicated to lifelong support of first-rate medical education efforts to insure that the science and art of medicine are passed on effectively to future generations of physicians. I shall be supportive of any patient's desire or efforts to seek alternate opinions on matters about which he or she may have doubts or questions. I believe that from the individual physician and from the profession each patient is owed every possible and reasonable safeguard.

• I, as a physician, shall charge only for my professional services and shall not profit financially in any other way as a result of the advice and care I render to my patients.

• I, as a member of my profession, recognize my responsibility to work for the development of policies and procedures which will safeguard and enhance the quality of medical care available to the community. I know I may help the community in making important health-related societal decisions by serving as an expert witness or consultant.

• I, as a member of my profession, recognize my responsibility to support the interest of the profession as a whole, and accept the fact that from time to time the profession's perceived interests may be at odds with other segments of the community.

• I, as a member of my profession, or as a citizen, may act in support of policies which may seem antithetical to groups of patients, but shall never allow those citizen or professional roles to interfere with my role as a physician caring for individual patients. Thus, I shall seek to acquire for my patients the best available care, even though as a citizen I might believe that a given modality of care might be too expensive for society to make available for all patients.

• I, as a physician and as a member of my profession, shall seek to provide disease prevention and health promotion information and services to my patients, my clients, and the public at large. When an individual is well and seeks the above services or advice, I shall provide them to the best of my ability and shall refer to the individual as a client. When an individual becomes diseased or is suffering in any way and seeks or needs my advice or services, she or he becomes my patient. The characteristics of these two important professional relationships are different and it can be seen that the same individual may become a patient, then a client, then a patient of the same physician over a relatively brief period of time. I shall take personal responsibility for the care of my patients, and I shall aid my clients to take personal care of themselves.

Now, Dr. Ross, you've asked me questions all day which I've answered with candor. It's my turn. What do you think of my new oath?

DR. ROSS: Well, in all frankness, Hippocrates, on first hearing I believe it says what needs to be said, but I have to agree with your editor. It'll never catch on, even if we can attach your name to it. It's too long, but also too modern. The old oath is like an antique chair; you really can't use it as a chair, but it gives you a sense of connection with the past. Your old oath connects all of us today to you in a more meaningful fashion than such a modern-sounding one.

HIPPOCRATES: But I didn't even write that old one, and I don't believe some of it.

DR. ROSS: True, but your antique oath containing so many things most doctors find currently irrelevant thereby allows the modern doctor to make up his or her own details. Sorry. It'll never sell.

HIPPOCRATES: I'm crushed. I've had it copyrighted and everything. Well, that's what I get for asking you questions. Now I'm depressed.

DR. ROSS: Oh, you of all people shouldn't be depressed by the truth! You asked my opinion as a kind of expert. I gave it truthfully as you requested. As with patient or client consultations (you see, I'm already using your terms) I must also tell you my opinion is only that—I have no scientific proof of my prognostication for your oath. So my prescription is that you should be hopeful and keep trying to promote your new oath, and we'll hope for a happy outcome. I shall do all I can to help you reach your goal; if I am confused about how to help, I shall seek other consultation; but, even in the event of failure, I'll stand beside you. It is a good oath.

HIPPOCRATES: Thank you, Dr. Ross, for your cheering speech. Like a good Greek physician you have become a friend to me . . . and in such a short time!

There is much more science and technology in medicine now, but the area of effective clinical practice that can be called "the art" is just as big and important as it used to be. Many modern doctors have lost sight of that. If that can be recovered, the young will always be attracted to the healing professions. Congratulations, Dr. Ross, on a life well lived.

I must go now, but please tell Dr. Bulger to get his book published if he can and not to despair—there are plenty of young Hippocrates out there, male and female.

DR. ROSS: Thank you, Hippocrates. It's been the chance of a lifetime for me and I'll tell Dr. Bulger your advice.

HIPPOCRATES: Thank you. One more thing. If the book is to be published, please tell Dr. Bulger he has my permission to print my new oath . . . with proper attribution of course!

DR. ROSS: Excuse me, Hippocrates, but I have a strange deep-down certainty that he already knows that . . . and it feels almost as if we're in the future somewhere. . . . I have one last question, though, if you can spare me a little more time.

HIPPOCRATES: Time is really not an issue any longer, Dr. Ross. Please go on.

DR. ROSS: Well, frankly, I interrupted you a little while ago when you were talking about why I was chosen to meet you and to participate in this dialogue.

HIPPOCRATES: I noticed, but I thought you were displaying your innate modesty in the face of my compliments.

DR. ROSS: No, I wasn't being modest. I was bothered by . . .

HIPPOCRATES: Well, when you interrupted me at that point I was explaining why you were chosen from among the many extraordinary and talented scientific physicians of the twentieth century. The reason was precisely because, in your dying, you, along with your family, elected to grow through the suffering and, as it happened, to share your experiences, thus teaching a wide array of others about suffering, about life and happiness . . . and about themselves. That's real healing, my friend.

DR. ROSS: Yes, but all that implies that I've finished dealing with death, and it has not been easy. It has been a hard and complicated thing, this living up to my suffering and death—much more demanding in some ways than going down suddenly with a heart attack or something, and I still may not succeed in carrying it off.

HIPPOCRATES: You have carried it off.

DR. ROSS: You mean . . . ?

HIPPOCRATES: Yes, Dr. Ross, these are the Elysian fields.

DR. ROSS: Well, I'll be. I always thought Mount Enterprise was heaven, but I'm surprised I wasn't more aware. Can it be such a narrow chasm to cross?

HIPPOCRATES: Griff, that's the way it seems to work when you have prepared well for your commencement. Welcome to life without time.

DR. ROSS: Thanks. It does feel pretty good—so far. Say, can you direct me to the library?

HIPPOCRATES: My word! You really are hungry for knowledge! Is it the *New England Journal* you miss?

DR. ROSS: In part . . . but, to tell the truth, I miss Pinky and the kids and I thought I could play with that machine you mentioned so that I could read their minds!

P.S. Shortly after this manuscript went to the editor, a letter was delivered postmarked "The Elysian fields" containing the following oath along with a brief note, which read as follows: "Dear Editor: Perhaps this is short enough! Sincerely, in the Spirit of Hippocrates."

The Oath of the Modern Hippocrates, 1987

• By all that I hold highest, I promise my patients competence, integrity, candor, personal commitment to their best interests, compassion, and absolute discretion and confidentiality within the law.

• I shall do by my patients as I would be done by; shall obtain consultation whenever I or they desire, shall include them to the extent they wish in all important decisions, and shall minimize suffering whenever a cure cannot be obtained, understanding that a dignified death is an important goal in everyone's life.

• I shall try to establish a friendly relationship with my patients and shall accept each one in a nonjudgmental manner, appreciating the validity and worth of different value systems and according to each person a full measure of human dignity.

• I shall charge only for my professional services and shall not profit financially in any other way as a result of the advice and care I render my patients.

• I shall provide advice and encouragement for my clients in their efforts to sustain their own health.

• I shall work with my profession to improve the quality of medical care and to improve the public health, but I shall not let any lesser public or professional consideration interfere with my primary commitment to provide the best and most appropriate care available to each of my patients.

• To the extent that I live by these precepts, I shall be a worthy physician.

# Notes on Contributors

Roger J. Bulger, M.D., F.A.C.P., President, the University of Texas Health Science Center at Houston (1978–), is also Professor of Medicine and Professor of Public Health. He has held a wide variety of administrative positions related to health professional education. For many years his publications were largely in the fields of microbiology, infectious disease and kidney disease; recently, however, he has published mostly in the areas of health policy, health promotion, and health services. In 1972 he edited the book *Hippocrates Revisited.*

Robert Coles, M.D., Research Psychiatrist, Harvard University Health Services, Cambridge, Massachusetts, has had an extraordinary career as a psychiatrist, author, educator, and lecturer. His studies on children are perhaps best known, but his interests are wide-ranging.

Ralph Crawshaw, M.D., Portland, Oregon, is a psychiatrist, author, and educator who has written widely and wisely on the nature of physicianhood.

Erik H. Erikson (deceased), Professor Emeritus of Human Development, Harvard University, Cambridge, Massachusetts, made major contributions to modern psychoanalytic thought, never failing to combine his brilliance and intellectual distinction with an uncommon sense of compassion and wisdom.

Guido Majno, M.D., Professor and Chairman, Department of Pathology, University of Massachusetts Medical Center, Worcester, Massachusetts, is an experimental pathologist and medical educator who has written *The Healing Hand,* a book praised as first-class anthropology.

Edmund D. Pellegrino, M.D., John Carroll Professor of Medicine and Medical Humanities, Georgetown University, Washington, D.C., has held numerous positions of responsibility and trust throughout a lifetime committed to medicine and higher education. Whether leading a medical school (SUNY at Stony Brook), a major hospital (Yale University Hospital), or a major university (Catholic University), he has continued to make significant contributions to the intellectual interface between medicine and philosophy.

Stanley J. Reiser, M.D., Ph.D., Griff T. Ross Professor of Humanities and Technology, the University of Texas Medical School, Houston, Texas, is a physician-historian and educator whose interest in technology development and human values has brought him international prominence.

Arnold S. Relman, M.D., Editor, *The New England Journal of Medicine,* Boston, Massachusetts, is an internist and medical editor who is one of the most influential physicians in the nation.

Dickinson W. Richards, M.D. (deceased), Lambert Professor Emeritus of Medicine, Columbia University College of Physicians and Surgeons, New York, New York, won the Nobel Prize in Medicine for his work on the use of cardiac catheterization. In later years Dr. Richards, a bona fide Greek scholar made seminal contributions to our understanding of the origins of Western medicine through his study of Hippocrates and his times.

David E. Rogers, M.D., former President, the Robert Wood Johnson Foundation, Princeton, New Jersey, and Dean of Johns Hopkins School of Medicine, and currently the Walsh McDermott Professor of Medicine at Cornell, is an internist and expert in infectious diseases who has become one of the most influential health policy makers in America. An accomplished sculptor as well, Dr. Rogers brings an unusually broad perspective to his thinking about medicine and biomedical science.

Lola Romanucci-Ross, Ph.D., Professor of Community and Family Medicine and Anthropology, University of California School of Medicine–San Diego, La Jolla, California, is a distinguished anthropologist with wide and varied experience. Among her books is *The Anthropology of Medicine: From Culture to Method* (with D. Moerman and L. Tancredi).

Howard M. Spiro, M.D., Professor of Medicine, Yale University School of Medicine, New Haven, Connecticut, is a well-known academic internist specializing in gastroenterology, with a particular interest in the art of medicine.

Laurence R. Tancredi, M.D., J.D., the University of Texas School of Public Health, Houston, Texas, directs the Health Law Program. A psychiatrist and lawyer with experience in health-policy-oriented positions at NIH and the Institute of Medicine of the National Academy of Medicine, Dr. Tancredi is a prodigious worker whose contributions to the literature cover an enormous range of issues located on the border between medical practice and the law.